GERIATRICS At Your FINGERTIPS

1998/99 EDITION

AUTHORS:

David B. Reuben, MD

George T. Grossberg, MD

Lorraine C. Mion, PhD, RN

James T. Pacala, MD, MS

Jane F. Potter, MD

Todd P. Semla, MS, PharmD, BCPS, FCCP

**PUBLISHED BY
EXCERPTA MEDICA, INC.
BELLE MEAD, NJ**

105 Raider Boulevard, Suite 101
Belle Mead, New Jersey 08502, USA

This publication was prepared by Excerpta Medica, Inc. at the direction of 1
American Geriatrics Society as a service to health care providers involved
the care of older persons. Partial funding for the development of this public
tion was provided by the John A. Hartford Foundation of New York City unde
grant to the American Geriatrics Society in support of the project (1998-200
entitled "Enhancing Geriatric Care Through Practicing Physician Education

The information in this publication was largely derived, with permission,
from the *Geriatrics Review Syllabus: A Core Curriculum in Geriatric Medicir*
Third Edition (Kendall/Hunt Publishing Company, 1996), a publication of th
American Geriatrics Society.

ISBN 444-01935-9
Library of Congress Catalog Card Number: 98-071029
Printed in the U.S.A.

TABLE OF CONTENTS

GERIATRICS *At Your* FINGERTIPS

Authors

David B. Reuben, MD
Director, Multicampus Program in Geriatric Medicine
   and Gerontology
Chief, Division of Geriatrics
Professor of Medicine
UCLA School of Medicine
Los Angeles, CA

George T. Grossberg, MD
Samuel W. Fordyce Professor
Chair, Department of Psychiatry
Director, Division of Geriatric Psychiatry
St. Louis University School of Medicine
St. Louis, MO

Lorraine C. Mion, PhD, RN
Director, Nursing Research
Cleveland Clinic Foundation
Cleveland, OH

James T. Pacala, MD, MS
Associate Professor
Program in Geriatrics
Department of Family Practice and Community Health
University of Minnesota Medical School
Minneapolis, MN

Jane F. Potter, MD
Chief, Section of Geriatrics and Gerontology
Department of Internal Medicine
Professor of Medicine
University of Nebraska Medical Center
Omaha, NE

Todd P. Semla, MS, PharmD, BCPS, FCCP
Clinical Pharmacology Unit
Evanston Hospital
Evanston, IL
Clinical Assistant Professor
Section of Geriatric Medicine
College of Medicine
University of Illinois at Chicago
Chicago, IL

INTRODUCTION

Geriatrics At Your Fingertips is designed to be a ready reference guide that provides immediate access to specific information needed to care for older persons in all health care settings. Within this guide are geriatric assessment instruments, specific recommended diagnostic tests for common clinical problems, and management strategies, including nonpharmacologic and pharmacologic therapy. To facilitate prescribing medications appropriately, generic and trade names are provided, as well as information on dosages, how the drug is metabolized or excreted, and how the drug is supplied. Frequently, we have included comparison tables that indicate specific cautions to be observed when using medication in older persons. The guide is organized by chapters similar to those found in the American Geriatric Society's (AGS) Geriatrics Review Syllabus; however, most users will find it more convenient to locate specific information by searching the index.

Although the authors have attempted to provide extensive clinical information, the guide is not all-inclusive. The guide does not attempt to explain in detail the rationale underlying the strategies presented. In many instances, these strategies have been derived from guidelines published by organizations such as the Agency for Health Care Policy and Research, the American Heart Association, and the American Diabetes Association. In other cases, no such guidelines exist and the strategies represent the best opinions of the authors and experts who have been asked to review the chapters. The guide is also not intended as a comprehensive pharmacopoeia. For some conditions, we provide only representative medications. We have also omitted medications that are infrequently used or are less appropriate for older persons. In other instances, we have included medications that are not the best choices for older persons, in general, but may benefit some individual patients and are in common usage. To keep the guide concise enough to be easily portable, references (except for some published guidelines) have not been provided; however, many are available from the organizations mentioned or can be found in the AGS *Geriatrics Review Syllabus*.

In preparing this first edition, we have had to make some decisions about the size and content of the text. We welcome specific comments, which should be addressed to the AGS, about the format and content of *Geriatrics At Your Fingertips* that may guide the preparation of future editions.

The editors are particularly grateful to Nancy Renick and Patricia Connelly at AGS, who have served vital roles in creating this book. We would also like to thank the following persons who have reviewed portions of the text that lie within their expertise:

Chris Costas, MD
Catherine Dubeau, MD
Bruce Ferrell, MD
John Fitzgerald, MD
Gail Greendale, MD
Bevra Hahn, MD
Donald Hay, MD
Thomas V. Jones, MD
Fran E. Kaiser, MD

Brenda K. Keller, MD
Patricia Morrow, MS
Lauren Nathan, MD
Anne Peters, MD
Elizabeth Reed, MD
Gary Rubin, PhD
Molly Sammon, RN
Ajay Singla, MD
Mary Tinetti, MD
James Webster, MD

Abbreviations of organizations whose guidelines have been the basis of parts of specific chapters:

Advisory Committee on Immunization Practices (ACIP)
Agency for Health Care Policy and Research (AHCPR)
American College of Gastroenterology (ACG)
American College of Obstetrics and Gynecology (ACOG)
American College of Rheumatology (ACR)
American Diabetes Association (ADA)
American Geriatrics Society (AGS)
American Heart Association (AHA)
American Psychiatric Association (APA)
American Thoracic Society (ATS)
American Thyroid Association (ATA)
National Heart, Lung, and Blood Institute (NHLBI)
US Preventive Services Task Force (USPSTF)
World Health Organization (WHO)

Abbreviations used in text:

ACEI - angiotensin-converting enzyme inhibitor
ADL - activities of daily living
B - biliary excretion
BID - twice a day
BP - blood pressure
BPH - benign prostatic hyperplasia
BUN - blood urea nitrogen
CBC - complete blood count
CHF - congestive heart failure
CNS - central nervous system
COPD - chronic obstructive pulmonary disease
CrCl - creatinine clearance
CT - computed tomography
CVA - stroke (cerebrovascular accident)
CXR - chest x-ray
DSM - *Diagnostic and Statistical Manual of Mental Disorders**
DVT - deep venous thrombosis

* *Diagnostic and Statistical Manual of Mental Disorders*, Fourth Edition. Washington, DC: American Psychiatric Association; 1994.

EKG - electrocardiogram
EPS - extrapyramidal symptoms
FDA - Food and Drug Administration
GAD - generalized anxiety disorder
GFR - glomerular filtration rate
GI - gastrointestinal
GU - genitourinary
HDL - high-density lipoprotein
HTN - hypertension
IADL - instrumental activities of daily living
IM - intramuscular
IV - intravenous
K - metabolized/excreted by kidney
L - metabolized/excreted by liver
LDL - low-density lipoprotein
LFTs - liver function tests
LVH - left ventricular hypertrophy
MAOIs - monoamine oxidase inhibitors
MI - myocardial infarction
MMSE - Mini-Mental State Examination
MRI - magnetic resonance imaging
Na - sodium
NPO - nothing by mouth
NS - normal saline
NSAIDs - nonsteroidal anti-inflammatory drugs
OCD - obsessive-compulsive disorder
OTC - over the counter
PE - pulmonary embolism
PNS - peripheral nervous system
po - by mouth
PPD - purified protein derivative
prn - as needed
PSA - prostate specific antigen
PTH - parathyroid hormone
q - every
qd - once daily, every day
qod - every other day
SC - subcutaneously
SSRIs - selective serotonin reuptake inhibitors
TCAs - tricyclic antidepressants
TD - tardive dyskinesia
TIA - transient ischemic attacks
TID - three times a day
TSH - thyroid-stimulating hormone (thyrotropin)
T $^1/_2$ - half-life
UA - urinalysis
WSR - Westergren sedimentation rate

Drug brand names are italicized in parentheses.
Drug formulations are in brackets.

AGE-RELATED PHYSIOLOGIC CHANGES AND FORMULAS

Table 1. Conversions

Temperature	Liquid	Weight
F = (1.8) C + 32	1 fluid dram = 4 mL	1 pound = 0.453 kg
C = (F-32) (1.8)	1 fluid ounce = 30 mL	1 kilogram = 2.2 lb
	1 teaspoon = 5 mL	1 ounce = 30 g
	1 tablespoon = 15 mL	1 grain = 60 mg

Table 2. Changes in Laboratory Values with Aging

Lab	Direction and Magnitude of Change
Hematologic	
Fibrinogen	↑
Clotting factors VII, VIII	↑↑
D-dimers	↑↑
ESR	↑↑
Arterial Blood Gases	
PaO$_2$	↓ (3 mm Hg/decade)
Chemistries	
Total protein	↓
Albumin	↓
Uric acid	↓
Alkaline phosphatase	↑
Postprandial glucose	↑ (5 mg/dL/decade at 2 hr)

Table 3. Key Physiologic Changes

Parameter	Impact
Hepatic clearance:	↓ Phase I — ↑ Drug half-life
Renal elimination:	↓ Renal blood flow
	↓ Tubular secretion
	↓ Glomerular filtration rate
Impaired thermal regulation	↑ Hypo-hyperthermia
	Blunted febrile response
Alterations helper T-cell function	↑ Infections
↓ Antibody-mediated response	↑ Autoimmune disorders
↓ Thymic hormones	
Changes in cytokine system	Uncertain

Formulas

Alveolar-arterial oxygen gradient = A-a = $148 - 1.2(PaCO_2) - PaO_2$
[normal = 10–20 mm Hg, breathing room air at sea level]

Calculated osmolality = 2Na + glucose/18 + BUN/2.8 + ethanol/4.6 + isopropanol/6 + methanol/3.2 + ethylene glycol/6.2 [norm 280–295]

Golden rules of arterial blood gases
(1) PCO$_2$ change of 10 corresponds to a pH change of 0.08.
(2) pH change of 0.15 corresponds to base excess change of 10 mEq/L.

Creatinine clearance = $\dfrac{\text{IBW}(140 - \text{age})(0.85 \text{ if female})}{(72)(\text{stable creatinine})}$
[normal >80]

Body Mass Index (BMI) = $\dfrac{\text{weight in kg}}{(\text{height in meters})^2}$ = $\dfrac{\text{weight in lbs}}{(\text{height in inches})^2}$ x 704.5

Ideal body weight: Male = 50 kg + (2.3 kg)(each inch of height >5 feet)
(IBW)   Female = 45.5 kg + (2.3 kg)(each inch of height >5 feet)

Partial pressure of oxygen, arterial (PaO_2) while breathing room air:
    60 years >80 mm Hg
    70 years >70 mm Hg
    80 years >60 mm Hg
    90 years >50 mm Hg

WSR (Westergren sedimentation rate):
    Women = (age + 10)/2
    Men = age/2

Table 4. Motor Function by Nerve Roots			
Level	**Motor Function**	**Level**	**Motor Function**
C4	Spontaneous breathing	L1/L2	Hip flexion
C5	Shoulder shrug	L3	Hip adduction
C6	Elbow flexion	L4	Hip abduction
C7	Elbow extension	L5	Great toe dorsiflexion
C8/T1	Finger flexion	S1/S2	Foot plantar flexion
T1-T12	Intercostal abdominal muscles	S2-S4	Rectal tone

Lumbosacral Nerve Root Compression

Root	Motor	Sensory	Reflex
L4	Quadriceps	Medial foot	Knee-jerk
L5	Dorsiflexors	Dorsum of foot	Medial hamstring
S1	Plantarflexors	Lateral foot	Ankle-jerk

Dermatomes

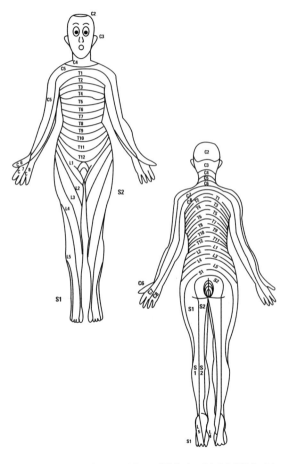

Source: *The Tarascon Pocket Pharmacopoeia.* Tarascon Publishing; Loma Linda, Calif. 1997:7. Permission to reprint.

APPROACH TO THE PATIENT

Dimensions of Assessment*

Dimension	Method	See Page No.
Frequently assessed:		
Medical status	History, physical examination, laboratory tests	7
Medications	Med Hx ("brown bag method")	16
Cognitive status	Mini-Mental State Examination	126
Functional status	Activities of Daily Living/IADL	127, 128
Social/financial status	Social history	
Emotional status	Geriatric Depression Scale (GDS)	129
Physical status	Physical evaluation	7
Balance and gait	Physical evaluation, POAM scale	131–133
Nutrition	Dietary history	32
Dentition	Dental examination	10–12
Environmental hazards	Home evaluation	34–36

*See "Assessment Instruments," p 126.

Review of Systems

Make sure to inquire about: functional change over past year or since last visit; medication use (see "Pharmacotherapy and Appropriate Prescribing," p 15); weight change; fatigue; dizziness; falls; sleep patterns; cardiovascular system such as chest pain, shortness of breath, or claudication; urinary patterns, especially incontinence; bowel patterns, especially constipation; hearing or visual changes; musculoskeletal stiffness or pain.

Physical Examination

Make sure to check: Height and weight, orthostatic blood pressure and pulse, skin integrity (all surfaces), visual acuity, hearing.

PREOPERATIVE AND PERIOPERATIVE CARE

Preoperative Care Checklist

1. Cardiac risk assessment – Assess patient for risk of perioperative cardiac complications (myocardial infarction, pulmonary edema, cardiac arrest): (1) Collect variables from the Modified Cardiac Risk Index (see **Table 5**, p 8); (2) If surgery is emergent, proceed directly to surgery; (3) If surgery is nonemergent, apply algorithm on **Table 6**, p 9.

2. Pulmonary risk assessment – Assess risk factors for pulmonary complications (respiratory failure, pneumonia, atelectasis). Spirometry has not been shown to be useful in risk assessment.

Table 5. Modified Cardiac Risk Index	
Variable	**Points**
Coronary artery disease	
Myocardial infarction <6 months earlier	10
Myocardial infarction >6 months earlier	5
Canadian Cardiovascular Society angina classification II	
Class III	10
Class IV	20
Alveolar pulmonary edema	
Within 1 week	10
Ever	5
Suspected critical aortic stenosis	20
Arrhythmias	
Rhythm other than sinus or sinus plus atrial premature beats on electrocardiogram	5
>5 premature ventricular contractions on electrocardiogram	5
Poor general medical status, defined as any of the following: PO_2 < 60 mm Hg, PCO_2 >50 mm Hg, K^+ level <3 mmol/L, blood urea nitrogen level >50 mg/dL (18 mmol/L), creatinine level >3 mg/dL (260 mmol/L), bedridden	5
Age >70 years	5
Emergency surgery	10

II = Canadian Cardiovascular Society classification of angina; III = angina with walking 1 to 2 level blocks or climbing 1 flight of stairs or less at a normal pace; IV = inability to perform any physical activity without development of angina.
Source: Detsky AS, Abrams HB, McLaughlin JR, et al. Predicting cardiac complications in patients undergoing non-cardiac surgery. *J Gen Intern Med.* 1986;1:211–219. Permission to reprint.

<u>Risk factors</u>: Increasing age; abnormal chest x-ray; and preoperative bronchodilator use, increasing American Society of Anesthesiologists (ASA) class (I – healthy; II – mild systemic disease or age >80; III – severe systemic disease; IV – life-threatening systemic disease; V – moribund).
<u>Procedures</u> associated with pulmonary complications are coronary artery bypass grafting and major abdominal operations.
<u>Postoperative</u> complications are minimized by incentive spirometry, coughing, and early ambulation.

3. Other assessments
<u>Cognitive status</u>: Unrecognized dementia is a risk factor for postoperative delirium. Measure preoperative cognitive status with MMSE (see p 126).
<u>Nutritional status</u>: Poor nutritional status can impair wound healing. Measure height, weight, serum albumin.
<u>Routine laboratory tests</u>: Recommend: Hemoglobin/hematocrit, electrolytes, creatinine, BUN, EKG, CXR, albumin. Optional: CBC, platelets, ABG, PT, PTT.
<u>Advance directives</u>: Establish or update.

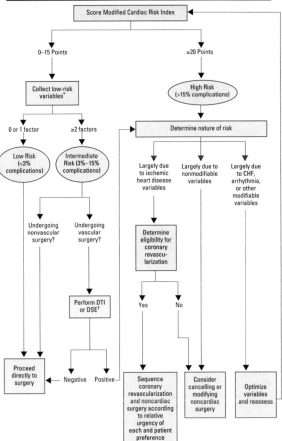

Table 6. Coronary Risk Assessment of Nonemergent, Noncardiac Surgery

Score Modified Cardiac Risk Index

0–15 Points → Collect low-risk variables*

≥20 Points → High Risk (>15% complications)

0 or 1 factor → Low Risk (<3% complications)

≥2 factors → Intermediate Risk (3%–15% complications)

Low Risk → Undergoing nonvascular surgery?

Intermediate Risk → Undergoing vascular surgery? → Perform DTI or DSE† → Negative / Positive

Proceed directly to surgery

High Risk → Determine nature of risk

Largely due to ischemic heart disease variables → Determine eligibility for coronary revascularization → Yes / No

Largely due to nonmodifiable variables

Largely due to CHF, arrhythmia, or other modifiable variables

Sequence coronary revascularization and noncardiac surgery according to relative urgency of each and patient preference

Consider cancelling or modifying noncardiac surgery

Optimize variables and reassess

*Low-risk variables are: Age >70 years, history of angina, diabetes mellitus, Q waves on EKG, history of MI, ST-segment ischemic abnormalities on resting EKG, hypertension with severe LVH, history of CHF.
†DTI = dipyridamole thallium imaging; DSE = dobutamine stress echocardiography.
Source: Adapted from American College of Physicians: Clinical Guideline, Part 1. Guidelines for assessing and managing perioperative risk from coronary artery disease associated with major noncardiac surgery. *Ann Intern Med.* 1997;127:309–312. Permission to reprint.

4. Perioperative management

   β-Blocker use: Patients with diagnosed coronary artery disease (CAD) or with >2 risk factors for CAD (male gender, hypertension, smoking, diabetes, dyslipidemia, obesity, family history, sedentary lifestyle) should receive perioperative atenolol, unless heart rate is <55 beats/min.; SBP <100; or the patient has asthma, CHF, or third degree heart block. Give two doses of atenolol IV, 5 mg administered over 5 minutes, the first 30 minutes before surgery, the second immediately after surgery. Following surgery, begin atenolol 50–100 mg po qd until discharge.

   DVT prophylaxis: General surgery: Elastic stockings plus low-dose unfractionated heparin (LDUH), 5,000 units SC 2 hours before surgery and q12h after surgery. For higher risk, consider LDUH q8h, low-molecular-weight heparin (LMWH), (enoxaparin [Lovenox] 30 mg SC q12h), and/or the use of intermittent pneumatic compression (IPC) devices. Total hip replacement: LMWH or warfarin (adjust INR 2.0 to 3.0) or dose-adjusted heparin. Total knee replacement: LMWH or IPC. Surgical hip fracture repair: LMWH or warfarin + IPC.

   Monitor common problems: Malnutrition: See "Malnutrition," p 32. Confusion: See p 18. Polypharmacy: Review medications daily. Skin breakdown: See "Pressure Ulcers," p 37. Rehabilitation: Encourage early mobility.

ENDOCARDITIS PROPHYLAXIS
(AMERICAN HEART ASSOCIATION GUIDELINES)

Antibiotic Prophylaxis (AP) Recommended (See Table 7, p 11)

Cardiac conditions requiring AP. High-risk category: Prosthetic heart valves, previous endocarditis, surgical systemic pulmonary shunts. Moderate-risk category: Acquired valvular dysfunction (eg, rheumatic heart disease), hypertrophic cardiomyopathy, mitral valve prolapse with valvular regurgitation and/or thickened leaflets, most congenital heart malformations.

Procedures warranting AP.

- Dental: Extractions, periodontal, implants and reimplants, root canals, subgingival placement of antibiotic fibers or strips, initial placement of orthodontic bands but not brackets, intraligamentary local anesthetic injections, teeth cleaning where bleeding is expected.
- Respiratory tract: Tonsillectomy and/or adenoidectomy, rigid bronchoscopy, surgery involving respiratory mucosa.
- Gastrointestinal tract: Esophageal varices sclerotherapy, esophageal stricture dilation, endoscopic retrograde cholangiography with biliary obstruction, biliary tract surgery, surgery involving intestinal mucosa.
- Genitourinary tract: Prostatic surgery, cystoscopy, urethral dilation.

AP Not Recommended

Cardiac conditions not requiring AP. Previous coronary artery bypass graft surgery; mitral valve prolapse without valvular regurgitation; physiologic, functional, or innocent heart murmurs; previous rheumatic fever without valvular dysfunction; cardiac pacemakers; implanted defibrillators; isolated secundum atrial septal defect, surgical repair of atrial or ventricular septal defect.

Procedures not warranting AP.

- Dental: Restorative dentistry, local anesthetic injections, intracanal endodontic treatment, rubber dam placement, suture removal, placement of removable prosthodontic or orthodontic appliances, oral impressions, fluoride treatments, oral radiographs, orthodontic appliance adjustment.
- Respiratory tract: Endotracheal intubation, flexible bronchoscopy (AP optional for high-risk patients), ear tube insertion.
- Gastrointestinal tract (AP optional for high-risk patients): Transesophageal echocardiography, endoscopy.
- Genitourinary tract: Vaginal hysterectomy (AP optional for high-risk patients), urethral catheterization of uninfected tissue.
- Other: Cardiac catheterization, balloon angioplasty.

Table 7. Endocarditis Prophylaxis Regimens

Situation	Regimen
Dental, oral, respiratory tract, or esophageal procedures	
Standard general prophylaxis	Amoxicillin 2.0 g po 1 hr before procedure
Unable to take oral medications	Ampicillin 2.0 g IM or IV ≤30 minutes before procedure
Allergic to penicillin	Clindamycin 600 mg or cephalexin 2.0 g or cefadroxil 2.0 g or azithromycin 500 mg or clarithromycin 500 mg po 1 hr before procedure
Allergic to penicillin and unable to take oral medications	Clindamycin 600 mg or cefazolin 1.0 g IM or IV ≤30 minutes before procedure
Genitourinary or gastrointestinal procedures	
High-risk patients	Ampicillin 2.0 g IM or IV + gentamicin 1.5 mg/kg IV/IM (not to exceed 120 mg) ≤30 minutes before procedure; 6 hrs later, ampicillin 1.0 g IM/IV or amoxicillin 1.0 g po
High-risk patients allergic to ampicillin/amoxicillin	Vancomycin 1.0 g IV over 1–2 hr + gentamicin 1.5 mg/kg IV/IM (not to exceed 120 mg); complete injection/infusion ≤30 minutes before procedure
Moderate-risk patients	Amoxicillin 2.0 g po 1 hr before procedure or ampicillin 2.0 g IM/IV ≤30 minutes before procedure
Moderate-risk patients allergic to ampicillin/amoxicillin	Vancomycin 1.0 g IV over 1–2 hr; complete infusion ≤30 minutes before procedure

Source: Dajani AS, Taubert KA, Wilson W, et al. Prevention of bacterial endocarditis: Recommendations by the American Heart Association. *JAMA.* 1997;277:1794–1801. Reprinted with permission.

AP FOR DENTAL PATIENTS WITH TOTAL JOINT REPLACEMENTS (TJR): Recommendations by the American Dental Association and American Academy of Orthopaedic Surgeons.

Conditions requiring AP for patients with TJR undergoing dental procedures: Inflammatory arthropathies (eg, rheumatoid arthritis, systemic lupus erythematosus); disease-, drug-, or radiation-induced immunosuppression; type 1 diabetes mellitus; first 2 years following joint replacement; previous prosthetic joint infection; malnourishment; hemophilia.

Conditions not requiring AP for patients with TJR undergoing dental procedures: Patients >2 years post-TJR who do not have one of the above conditions; patients with pins, plates, or screws.

Dental procedures warranting AP for TJR patients are the same as those listed for endocarditis (see p 10).

Suggested prophylactic regimens (all given 1 hour before procedure):
- Not allergic to penicillin: Amoxicillin, cephalexin, or cephradine 2.0 g po.
- Not allergic to penicillin and unable to take oral medications: Ampicillin 2.0 g or cefazolin 1.0 g IM/IV.
- Allergic to penicillin: Clindamycin 600 mg po.
- Allergic to penicillin and unable to take oral medications: Clindamycin 600 mg IV.

Source: American Dental Association/American Academy of Orthopaedic Surgeons. Antibiotic prophylaxis for dental patients with total joint replacements. *JADA*. 1997;128:1004–1007. Reprinted with permission.

Prevention

Table 8. Recommendations for Primary and Secondary Disease Prevention Activities in Persons Aged 65 and Over

Preventive Activity	Endorsed by USPSTF*	Not Endorsed by USPSTF for All Older Adults, but Recommended in Selected Patients or by Other Professional Organizations
Primary Prevention		
Aspirin chemoprophylaxis		X
Blood pressure screening	X	
Cholesterol screening		X
Obesity (height and weight)	X	
Smoking cessation	X	
Diabetes screening		X
Influenza immunization	X	
Pneumonia immunization	X	
Tetanus immunization	X	
Hormone replacement therapy		X
Secondary Prevention		
Mammography/clinical breast examination	X†	
Breast self-examination		X
Annual skin examination		X
Pap smear	X‡	
Fecal occult blood testing	X	
Sigmoidoscopy	X	
Prostate specific antigen (PSA)		X
Visual impairment screening	X	
Hearing impairment screening	X	
Cognitive impairment screening		X
Bone densitometry		X

* US Preventive Services Task Force. *Guide to Clinical Preventive Services.* 2nd ed. Baltimore: Williams and Wilkins; 1996.
† Mammograms to age 70 are virtually universally recommended; many organizations, including the USPSTF, recommend that mammography should be continued in women over 70 who have a reasonable life expectancy.
‡ Most organizations recommend stopping pap smear testing at age 65 if the patient has had no disease detected on routine screening up until that age. See "Women's Health," p 111.

ELDER ABUSE

Risk Factors for Abuse of the Elderly

- Poor health and functional impairment in the elderly
- Cognitive impairment in the elderly
- Substance abuse or mental illness on the part of the abuser
- Dependence of the abuser on the victim
- Shared living arrangement
- External factors causing stress
- Social isolation
- History of violence

Source: Lachs MS, Pillemer K. *N Engl J Med.* 1995;332(7):437–443. Copyright 1995 Massachusetts Medical Society. All rights reserved. Reprinted with permission.

Presentations That Suggest Abuse or Neglect of an Elderly Patient

- Delays between an injury or illness and the seeking of medical attention
- Disparity in histories from the patient and the suspected abuser
- Implausible or vague explanations provided by either party
- Frequent visits to the emergency room for exacerbations of chronic disease despite a plan for medical care and adequate resources
- Presentation of a functionally impaired patient without his or her designated caregiver
- Laboratory findings that are inconsistent with the history provided

Source: Lachs MS, Pillemer K. *N Engl J Med.* 1995;332(7):437–443. Copyright 1995 Massachusetts Medical Society. All rights reserved. Reprinted with permission.

Specific Questions Regarding an Abusive Situation

Many abuse victims can be identified simply by asking patients direct questions such as the following:
- Has anyone at home ever hurt you?
- Are you afraid of anyone in your family?
- Has anyone ever scolded or threatened you?
- Are you receiving enough care at home?

Source: Jones JS. Abuse and neglect. In: Sanders AB, ed. *Emergency Care of the Elder Person.* St. Louis, Mo: Beverly Cracom Publications: 181. Reprinted with permission.

Exercise Prescription
Before receiving an exercise prescription (EP), patients should be screened for:
- Musculoskeletal problems: Decreased flexibility, muscular rigidity, weakness, pain, ill-fitting shoes.
- Cardiac disease: Consider stress test if sedentary person with ≥2 cardiac risk factors (male gender, hypertension, smoking, diabetes, dyslipidemia,

obesity, family history, sedentary lifestyle) is beginning a vigorous exercise program.

The EP should specify short- and long-term goals. Components of the EP should include:

- Flexibility: Static stretching; daily, >15 seconds per muscle group.
- Endurance: Walking, cycling, swimming at 50%–75% of maximum HR; 3–4x/wk; goal of 20–30 minutes in duration.
- Strength: Muscle resistance (weight training); 3 sets (8–15 repetitions) per muscle group 2–3x/wk.
- Balance: Tai chi, dance, postural awareness; 1–3x/wk.

NURSING HOME ASSESSMENT

Admissions Checklist

1. History, physical, labs as needed; PPD.
2. Determine functional status: ADL, IADL, MMSE, depression scale.
3. Review medications (correlate to active diagnoses).
4. Identify medical conditions — review old records.
5. Establish relationships — resident, family, staff.
6. Establish advance directives.
7. Formulate problem list.
8. Formulate plan.

Scheduled Visit Checklist

1. Evaluate patient for interval functional change.
2. Check vital signs, weight, labs, consultant reports since last visit.
3. Review medications (correlate to active diagnoses).
4. Sign orders.
5. Address nursing staff concerns.
6. Write a SOAP note.
7. Revise problem list as needed.
8. Update advance directives at least yearly.
9. Update resident; update family member(s) as needed.

Health Maintenance

Yearly: Functional status, mini-mental status, depression screen, vision, hearing, dental, podiatric, history, physical, creatinine, hemoglobin, TSH in women. Other labs and preventive procedures to be decided individually.
Monthly: Weight, vital signs.
Ongoing: Skin integrity, accident prevention, infection control.
Immunizations: *Flu vaccine* — once/yr in the fall months; (*Pneumovax*) — once at age 65; *tetanus* — every 10 years.

PHARMACOTHERAPY AND APPROPRIATE PRESCRIBING

Table 9. Age-Associated Changes in Pharmacokinetics and Pharmacodynamics

Parameter	Age Effect	Disease/Factor Effect	Prescribing Implication
Absorption	Rate and extent are usually unaffected	Achlorhydria, concurrent medications, tube feedings	Drug-drug and drug-food interactions are more likely to alter absorption
Distribution	Increase in fat:water ratio. Decreased plasma protein, particularly albumin	CHF, ascites and other conditions will ↑ body water	Fat-soluble drugs have a larger volume of distribution. Highly protein-bound drugs will have a greater (active) free concentration
Metabolism	Decreases in liver mass and liver blood flow may ↓ drug metabolism	Smoking, genotype, concurrent drug therapy, alcohol and caffeine intake may have more effect than aging	Drugs with phase I metabolism affected (eg, diazepam, phenytoin, verapamil, antidepressants)
Elimination	Primarily renal. Age-related ↓ in GFR	Renal impairment with acute and chronic diseases. ↓ muscle mass results in ↓ creatinine production	Serum creatinine not a reliable measure of renal function; best to estimate creatinine clearance using the formula on page 5
Pharmaco-dynamics	Less predictable and often altered drug response at usual or lower concentrations	Drug-drug and drug-disease interactions may alter responses	Prolonged pain relief with morphine at lower doses. ↑ sedation and postural instability to benzo-diazepines. Altered sensitivity to β-blockers

Aggravating Factors

- Drug-food/nutrient interactions:
  - Physical interactions. Food or nutrients ↓ or ↑ drug absorption. Examples include products containing Mg^{++}, Ca^{++}, Fe^{++}, Al^{++}, or zinc can decrease the oral absorption of quinolone antibiotics, and tube feedings will ↓ the absorption of oral phenytoin.
  - Decreased drug effect. Food or nutritional supplements can alter the intended pharmacologic response. The best example of this is warfarin and vitamin K-containing foods.
  - Decreased oral intake or appetite. Drugs can alter the taste of food (dysgeusia) or decrease saliva production (xerostomia) making mastication and swallowing difficult. Examples of drugs associated with dysgeusia include captopril and clarithromycin. Drugs which can cause xerostomia include antihistamines, antidepressants, antipsy-chotics, clonidine, and diuretics.
- Drug-drug interactions: A drug's effect can be ↑ or ↓ by another drug because of impaired absorption (eg, sucralfate and ciprofloxacin), displacement from protein-binding sites (eg, warfarin and sulfonamides), inhibition or induction of metabolic enzymes, or by two or more drugs that have a similar pharmacologic effect (eg, potassium-sparing diuretics, potassium supplements, and angiotensin-converting enzyme inhibitors).

Table 10. Drug-Disease Interactions		
Disease	**Drugs**	**Adverse Effect**
Benign prostatic hyperplasia	Anticholinergics, calcium channel blockers, decongestants	Urinary retention
Cardiac conduction abnormalities	Verapamil, TCAs, β-blockers (all routes)	Heart block
COPD	β-Blockers (all routes), narcotic analgesics	Bronchoconstriction, respiratory depression
Chronic renal insufficiency	NSAIDs, contrast agents, aminoglycosides	Acute renal failure
CHF (systolic)	β-Blockers (all routes), verapamil	CHF exacerbation
Dementia	Anticholinergics, benzodiazepines, opiates, antidepressants, antiparkinsonian agents	Delirium
Diabetes mellitus	Diuretics, corticosteroids	Hyperglycemia
Angle-closure glaucoma	Anticholinergics	Acute ↑ in IOP
Hypertension	NSAIDs	Increased blood pressure
Hypokalemia	Digoxin	Cardiac arrhythmias
Hyponatremia	Oral hypoglycemics, diuretics, SSRIs, carbamazepine, antipsychotics	↓ Serum sodium
Peptic ulcer	NSAIDs	Upper GI bleeding
Postural hypotension	Diuretics, TCAs, MAOIs, vasodilators, antiparkinsonian agents	Syncope, falls, hip fracture

Source: Adapted from Parker BM, Cusack BJ. Pharmacology and appropriate prescribing. In: Reuben DB, Yoshikawa TT, Besdine RW, eds. *Geriatrics Review Syllabus: A Core Curriculum in Geriatric Medicine.* 3rd ed. Dubuque, Iowa; Kendall/Hunt Publishing Company for the American Geriatrics Society; 1996:33.

How to prescribe appropriately and avoid polypharmacy:

- Obtain a complete drug history. Be sure to ask about previous treatments and response as well as about other prescribers. Ask about allergies, OTC drugs, nutritional supplements, alternative medications, alcohol, tobacco, caffeine, and recreational drugs.
- Avoid prescribing before a diagnosis is made. Consider nondrug therapy. Eliminate drugs for which no diagnosis can be identified.
- Review medications regularly and before prescribing a new medication. Discontinue medications that have not had the intended response or are no longer needed. Monitor the use of prn and OTC drugs.
- Know the actions, adverse effect, and toxicity profiles of the medications you prescribe. Consider how these might interact or complement existing drug therapy.
- Start chronic drug therapy at a low dose and titrate dose based on tolerability and response. Use drug levels when available.
- Attempt to maximize dose before switching or adding another drug.
- Encourage compliance with therapy. Educate patient and/or caregiver about each medication, its regimen, the therapeutic goal, its cost, and potential adverse effects or drug interactions. Provide written instructions.
- Avoid using one drug to treat the side effects of another.
- Attempt to use one drug to treat two or more conditions.
- Avoid combination products.

- Communicate with other prescribers. Don't assume the patient will—they assume you do!
- Avoid using drugs from the same class or with similar actions (eg, alprazolam and zolpidem).

Management

Table 11. Drugs to Avoid in the Elderly	
Drug	**Potential Problems or Concerns**
Propoxyphene (*Darvon, Darvocet*) and combination products	Same side effects as narcotic analgesics, with analgesic action comparable to acetaminophen
Indomethacin (*Indocin, Indocin SR*)	CNS side effects more common in the elderly
Phenylbutazone (*Butazolidin*)	May produce serious hematological side effects
Pentazocine (*Talwin*)	CNS side effects (confusion, hallucinations), mixed agonist-antagonist
Trimethobenzamide (*Tigan*)	Better antiemetics are available; risk of extrapyramidal reactions
Methocarbamol (*Robaxin*), carisoprodol (*Soma*), cyclobenzaprine (*Flexeril*), chloroxazone (*Paraflex*), metoxalone (*Skelaxin*)	Poorly tolerated at effective doses, anticholinergic side effects, sedation, and weakness
Diazepam (*Valium*), flurazepam (*Dalmane*), chlordiazepoxide (*Librium*), and other long-acting benzodiazepines, combinations	Accumulation, sedation, increased risk of falls and fractures
Amitriptyline (*Elavil*), doxepin (*Sinequan*), chlordiazepoxide-amitriptyline (*Limbitrol*) and perphenazine-amitriptyline (*Triavil*)	The most sedating and anticholinergic of the tricyclic antidepressants; rarely the antidepressant of choice for the elderly
Meprobamate (*Miltown*)	Highly addictive and sedating; those on it for a long time may need to be withdrawn
Disopyramide (*Norpace, Norpace CR*)	Potent negative inotrope and strongly anticholinergic
Dipyridamole (*Persantine*)	Limited proven role; frequently causes orthostatic hypotension
Methyldopa (*Aldomet*), methyldopa/hydrochlorothiazide (*Aldoril*)	Better alternatives are available; may cause bradycardia and exacerbate depression
Reserpine (*Serpasil, Hydropres*)	Depression, impotence, sedation, and orthostatic hypotension
Chlorpropamide (*Diabinese*)	Prolonged half-life increases risk of hypoglycemia
Dicyclomine (*Bentyl*), hyoscyamine (*Levsin*), other GI antispasmodics	Highly anticholinergic; may cause toxicity
Chlorpheniramine (*Chlor-Trimeton*), diphenhydramine (*Benadryl*), hydroxyzine (*Atarax, Vistaril*), other antihistamines	Many antihistamines are highly anticholinergic and may cause toxicity; avoid use as hypnotics; use lowest possible dose to treat allergic reactions
Ergoloid mesylates (*Hydergine*), cyclandelate (*Cyclospasmol*)	Ineffective in the treatment of most dementias including Alzheimer's disease
Iron supplements	Limit dose to no more than 325 mg/d of ferrous sulfate; constipation offsets the limited increase in absorption
All barbiturates other than phenobarbital	Highly addictive; many side effects
Meperidine (*Demerol*)	Decreased renal clearance results in accumulation of neurotoxic metabolite (delirium and seizures); not very effective orally
Ticlopidine (*Ticlid*)	Not more effective than aspirin and more toxic; use only when aspirin allergy or intolerance

Source: Adapted from Beers MH. *Arch Intern Med*. 1997;157:1531–1536. Permission to reprint.

DELIRIUM

Diagnostic Criteria - *DSM-IV* - American Psychiatric Association
Delirium due to a general medical condition:

A. Disturbance of consciousness (ie, reduced clarity of awareness of environment) with reduced ability to focus, sustain, or shift attention.

B. A change in cognition (such as memory deficit, disorientation, language disturbance) or the development of a perceptual disturbance that is no better accounted for by a preexisting, established, or evolving dementia.

C. The disturbance develops over a short period of time (usually hours to days) and tends to fluctuate during the course of the day.

D. There is evidence from the history, physical examination, or laboratory findings that the disturbance is caused by the direct physiological consequences of a general medical condition.

Risk Factors
Preexisting cognitive impairment, advanced age, comorbid medical problems.

Evaluation
Delirium should be assumed to be reversible unless proven otherwise. Comprehensive evaluation should include a thorough review of medications, both prescribed and OTC (see below). Infection should be ruled out. A systematic evaluation to exclude medical causes (see below) should be conducted. Laboratory evaluation may include a CBC, chemistries (electrolytes, liver and renal function tests, serum calcium, and glucose), urinalysis, oxygen saturation, CXR, and EKG to further identify potential causes of delirium.

CAUSES OF DELIRIUM

Drugs
• Anticholinergic (eg, diphenhydramine), tricyclic antidepressants (eg, amitriptyline, imipramine), neuroleptics (eg, chlorpromazine, thioridazine).
• Benzodiazepines—acute toxicity or withdrawal.
• Alcohol—acute toxicity or withdrawal.
• Lithium.
• Cardiovascular (eg, digitalis, antihypertensives, antiarrhythmics).
• Gastrointestinal (eg, cimetidine, metoclopramide, ranitidine).
• Narcotic analgesics (especially meperidine).
• Anti-inflammatory agents.
• Diuretics.

Infections
• Urinary tract, respiratory, skin, and others.

Metabolic Disorders
• Electrolyte imbalance, hypo-/hyperglycemia, hypoxia, acute blood loss, end-organ failure (hepatic, renal).

Cardiovascular
• Arrhythmia, myocardial infarction, congestive heart failure, shock.

Neurologic
• TIA, CVA, head trauma, subdural hematoma, seizures, CNS infections, tumors.

POSTOPERATIVE STATES

Miscellaneous
• Sleep deprivation.
• Urinary retention.
• Fecal impaction.

Nonpharmacologic Management
• Identification and removal/treatment of underlying cause is most important.
• General supportive measures include:
  – Keep patient in quiet, well-lit room (night lights at night).
  – Avoid excessive noise, stimulation.
  – Allow familiar faces such as family members to be present at bedside for reassurance.
  – Provide orientation (eg, calendar, clock).
  – Correct sensory impairment (eg, vision, hearing).
  – Communicate in succinct, direct style.
  – Use physical restraints only as a last resort to maintain patient safety or to prevent patient from pulling out tubes and catheters.

Pharmacologic Management
For acute agitation/aggressivity accompanying delirium, use a high-potency neuroleptic such as haloperidol (*Haldol*) 0.5 to 2 mg po [0.5, 1, 2, 5, 10, 20, liquid 2 mg/mL] or IM. May also be given as slow IV push, and titrated upwards as needed. Patient may require up to 10–20 mg over 24 hours. Reevaluate every 30 minutes. Observe for development of extrapyramidal symptoms. Avoid low-potency neuroleptics, (eg, chlorpromazine, thioridazine) because of their anticholinergic properties.

If delirium is secondary to alcohol or benzodiazepine withdrawal, the use of a benzodiazepine such as lorazepam or alprazolam (see Chapter 17, Anxiety) in doses of 0.5–2 mg every 4–6 hours and thiamine, 100 mg po qd (if delirium secondary to alcohol), may be helpful. Since these agents themselves may be causes of delirium, gradual withdrawal and discontinuation are desirable.

DEMENTIA

DIAGNOSTIC CRITERIA – (*DSM-IV*)

Dementia Syndrome
• Multiple cognitive impairments – months to years.
• Memory impairment, language, judgment, executive function impairments.

- Functional decline (from previous functional/cognitive functioning).
- Not in context of delirium.

Dementia of the Alzheimer Type (DAT)
- Most common cause of progressive dementia – accounts for about 70% (including mixed).

Diagnostic Criteria – DAT
A. Multiple cognitive deficits manifested by both:
    1. Memory impairment (impaired ability to learn new information or to recall previously learned information) and
    2. One (or more) of the following cognitive disturbances:
        a. Aphasia (language disturbance)
        b. Apraxia (impaired ability to carry out motor activities despite intact motor functions)
        c. Agnosia (failure to recognize or identify objects despite intact sensory functions)
        d. Disturbance in executive function (eg, planning, organizing, sequencing, abstracting).
B. The cognitive deficits in A1 and A2 each cause significant impairment in social or occupational functioning and represent a significant decline from a previous level of functioning.
C. Gradual onset and continuing cognitive decline.
D. The cognitive deficits are not due to any of the following:
    1. Other CNS conditions that cause progressive deficits in memory and cognition (eg, cerebrovascular disease, Parkinson's disease, Huntington's disease, subdural hematoma, normal pressure hydrocephalus, brain tumor)
    2. Systemic conditions known to cause dementia (eg, hypothyroidism, B_{12} or folate deficiency, hypercalcemia, neurosyphilis, HIV infection)
    3. Substance-induced conditions.
E. The deficits do not occur exclusively during the course of a delirium.
F. The disturbance is not better accounted for by another mental disorder (eg, major depression, schizophrenia).

Evaluation of DAT
- History – obtained from family/other informant.
- Physical/neurologic examination.
- Mental status evaluation (eg, MMSE).
- Assessment of functional status.

Laboratory Testing
- CBC, TSH, B_{12}, serum calcium, liver and renal function tests, electrolytes, serologic test for syphilis. Potentially useful – CXR, EKG, UA, sed rate.

Neuroimaging if:
- Onset <60 yrs.
- Focal (unexplained) neurologic signs or symptoms.
- Abrupt onset or rapid decline (weeks to months).
- Predisposing conditions (eg, metastatic cancer or anticoagulants).

Source: Small GW, Rabins PV, Barry PB, et al. Diagnosis and Treatment of Alzheimer Disease and Related Disorders: Consensus Statement of the American Association for Geriatric Psychiatry, the Alzheimer's Association, and the American Geriatrics Society. *JAMA*. 1997;278:1363–1371. Permission to reprint.

Risk Factors for DAT
• Advanced age.
• Female sex.
• Family history.
• Down syndrome or family history of Down syndrome.
• Apo E status (Apo ε-4 – increased risk).

STAGES OF DAT

Early/Mild   Years 1–3 (From Onset of Symptoms)   MMSE: 22–28
• Disorientation for date.
• Naming difficulties (anomia).
• Recent recall problems.
• Mild difficulty copying figures.
• Decreased insight.
• Withdrawal – social.
• Irritability/mood change.
• Problems managing finances.

Middle/Moderate   Years 2–8   MMSE: 10–21
• Disoriented to date, place, perhaps time.
• Comprehension difficulties (aphasia).
• Impaired new learning.
• Getting lost in familiar areas.
• Impaired calculating skills.
• Delusions/agitation/aggressivity.
• Not cooking/shopping/banking.
• Restless/anxious/depressed.
• Problems with dressing/grooming.

Late/Severe   Years 6–12   MMSE: 0–9
• Nearly unintelligible verbal output.
• Remote memory gone.
• Unable to copy or write.
• Apraxia.
• No longer grooming/dressing.
• Incontinent.

Vascular Dementia (VaD) – *DSM-IV*
Second most common cause of progressive dementia.

Diagnostic Criteria
A. The development of multiple cognitive deficits manifested by both:
    1. Memory impairment
    2. One or more of the following cognitive disturbances:
        a. Aphasia

b. Apraxia
　　　c. Agnosia
　　　d. Disturbance in executive functioning.
B. 　Above cognitive deficits each cause significant impairment in social or occupational functioning and represent a significant decline from a previous level of functioning.
C. 　Focal neurologic signs and symptoms (eg, exaggeration of DTRs, extensor plantar response, pseudobulbar palsy, gait abnormalities, weakness of an extremity) or laboratory evidence of cerebrovascular disease (eg, multiple infarctions involving cortex and underlying white matter) that is judged to be etiologically related to the disturbance.
D. 　Deficits do not occur exclusively during the course of a delirium.

Modified Hachinski Ischemic Score*

	Absent	Present
Abrupt onset	0	2
Stepwise deterioration	0	1
Somatic complaints	0	1
Emotional incontinence	0	1
History or presence of hypertension	0	1
History of strokes	0	2
Focal neurologic signs	0	2
Focal neurologic symptoms	0	2

*A score that is ≥4 is suggestive of vascular dementia.
Source: Rosen WG, Terry RD, Fuld PA, et al. Pathologic verification of ischemic score in differentiation of dementias. *Ann Neurol.* Lippincott-Raven Publishers; New York. 1980;7:487. Reprinted with permission.

TREATMENT OF DAT

- **Psychiatric Sequelae**
  - Psychotic symptoms (eg, delusions/hallucinations) occur in about one third of patients with DAT; delusions may be accusatory (eg, people stealing things) or paranoid. Hallucinations are more commonly visual. Nonpharmacologic treatments include identifying and eliminating possible environmental triggers.

Pharmacologic interventions: (see **Table 12**, p 24) Must assess risk-benefit ratio of using neuroleptic. Use smallest effective doses, monitor for side effects (extrapyramidal symptoms, tardive dyskinesia) and attempt to discontinue neuroleptic as soon as feasible.

Neuroleptics of choice: High-potency traditional neuroleptic (eg, haloperidol – daily dose 0.5–2 mg), or novel agents (eg, risperidone 0.5–2 mg/day; olanzapine 2.5–10 mg/day). If patient in nursing home environment, remember OBRA regulations relative to use of neuroleptics (see Chapter 34).

- Depressive symptoms: Occur in up to 40% of DAT patients. May herald onset of DAT – an early marker. May cause rapid acceleration or decline

if untreated. Need to suspect if patient stops eating or withdraws. Nonpharmacologic approaches (eg, activities, support, encouragement) are helpful, but rule out contributors to depression (eg, medications, underlying medical problems).
Pharmacotherapy is effective. Avoid anticholinergic antidepressants. Use newer agents (eg, SSRIs, nefazodone, bupropion, mirtazapine).
• Agitation/aggressivity: Occurs in up to 80% of patients with DAT. A leading cause of nursing home admissions. Consider agitation in the context of delirium, depression, or psychosis. Consider pain as a trigger.

General Treatment Principles
• Identify and treat primary medical illnesses.
• Set realistic goals.
• Limit PRN medication use.
• Allow adequate therapeutic trial.
• Specify and quantify target behaviors.
• Maintain functioning.

Nonpharmacologic Approaches
• Behavioral techniques (eg, distraction).
• Environmental modification (eg, feeding, reduce stimulation).
• Group programs (eg, for sundowning).
• Sound (soothing music), touch (massage therapy), routines.
• Use of family members to calm/reassure patient.

Pharmacologic Treatment – General Principles
• Start low/go slow.
• Assess target symptoms and toxicity.
• Titrate dose upward until benefit or toxicity.
• Maintain efficacious dose that is nontoxic or subtoxic.
• Serum drug levels may be helpful.
• Every case is an empiric trial of symptomatic pharmacotherapy.

Treatment of DAT – Cognitive Dysfunction
• Cholinesterase inhibitors (see **Table 13,** p 25) can improve cognition and moderate course of DAT in selected patients.
• Best candidates for cholinesterase inhibitor therapy: Mild to moderate Alzheimer's disease; no medical contraindications; supervision available.
• Evaluation of response to cholinesterase inhibitors
  – Caregiver observations are important relative to behavior (alertness, initiative) and function (ADL).
  – Cognition — improved or stabilized (by caregivers report or test scores).

Caregiver Issues
Caregivers of dementia patients are at risk for decompensating themselves due to the stresses of caregiving. Depression in caregivers needs to be recognized and treated. The Alzheimer's Association (1-800-272-3900), with chapters throughout the United States, is an invaluable source of information and support for family caregivers.

Table 12. Agitation Treatment Guidelines

Symptom	Drug	Dose	Metabolism	Formulations	Caveat
Psychotic or acutely agitated/out of control	Haloperidol (*Haldol*) or thiothixene (*Navane*)	0.5–2 mg/day 2–4 mg/day	Hepatic Hepatic	[Tablets 0.5, 1, 2.5, 10, 20] [Liquid 2 mg/mL] [Injectable]	May need to give higher doses in emergency situations to get patient under control
Agitation in context of psychosis (nonacute)	Risperidone (*Risperdal*) Olanzapine (*Zyprexa*)	0.5–2 mg/day 2.5–10 mg/day	Hepatic Hepatic	[Tablets, 1, 2, 3, 4, liquid] [Tablets 2.5, 5, 7.5, 10]	
Agitation in context of depression	SSRI (eg, sertraline [*Zoloft*] or nefazodone [*Serzone*])	25–100 mg/day 100–300 mg/day	Hepatic Hepatic	Tablets [Tablets 100, 150, 200, 250]	
Anxiety/mild-to-moderate irritability	Trazodone (*Desyrel*)	50–100 mg/day	Hepatic	[Tablets 50, 100, 150, 300]	Small divided daytime dosage and large bedtime dosage/watch for sedation and orthostasis
	Buspirone (*Buspar*)	30–60 mg/day	Hepatic	[Tablets 5, 10, 15, 30]	Can be given bid 2–4 weeks for optimal effect
Significant agitation or aggressivity	Divalproex sodium (*Depakote*)	500–1500 mg/day	Hepatic	[Tablets 125, 250, 500, syrup 250 mg/mL] Sprinkles	Can monitor serum levels, usually well tolerated
	Carbamazepine (*Tegretol*)	300–600 mg/day	Hepatic	[Tablets 100, 200] [Suspension 100/5 mL]	Monitor serum levels, periodic CBCs, platelet counts secondary to agranulocytosis risk Beware of multiple drug-drug interactions
Sexually aggressive/impulse-control symptoms in males	Estrogen (*Premarin*) or progestin (*Depo-Provera*)	0.625–1.25 mg/day 100 mg/IM weekly		[Tablets 0.3, 0.625, 0.9, 1.25, 2.5] Injectable	

24

	Table 13. Cholinesterase Inhibitors	
	Tacrine (*Cognex*)	Donepezil* (*Aricept*)
Dosing	10–40 mg qid	5–10 mg qd
Formulations	[10, 20, 30, 40]	[5, 10]
Labs	ALT levels	None required
Lab abnormalities	Increased ALT levels in 30%	None
Side effects	Mostly GI	Minimal
Dropout rate	High	Low

* Donepezil is given once daily at a starting dose of 5 mg. Some patients require 10 mg qd for optimal effect. Most clinicians recommend a 90-day trial at 5 mg. If no response, an increase to 10 mg qd can be tried. Side effects increase with higher dosing. Possible side effects of cholinesterase inhibitors include nausea, vomiting, diarrhea, dyspepsia, anorexia, weight loss, leg cramps, bradycardia, and agitation.

URINARY INCONTINENCE

Definition
Loss of urine control, sufficient to be a problem because of genitourinary pathology, age-related changes, comorbid conditions, environmental obstacles, or some combination of these. Urinary incontinence (UI) is not a normal part of aging.

Classification
• Transient: DIAPPERS mnemonic
   Delirium or confusional state; **I**nfection; **A**trophic vaginitis/urethritis; **P**harmacologic agents that impair cognition, mobility, fluid balance, or sphincter function; **P**sychological disorders, depression, severe psychosis; **E**xcessive urine output (glycosuria, hypercalcemia, diuretics, CHF, etc.); **R**estricted mobility from acute or chronic disorders; **S**tool impaction.

Established
• Urge-detrusor muscle overactivity (uninhibited bladder contractions); small to large volume loss; may be idiopathic or associated with CNS lesions or bladder irritation from infection, stones, tumors.
• Stress: Failure of sphincter mechanisms to remain closed during bladder filling (often due to insufficient pelvic support in women and sometimes after prostate surgery in men); loss occurs with increased intra-abdominal pressure.
• Overflow: Impaired detrusor contractility or bladder outlet obstruction. Outlet obstruction: BPH in men, cancer, stricture; in women, prior incontinence surgery or large cystocele. Impaired contractility: Chronic outlet obstruction, diabetes, vitamin B_{12} deficiency, tabes dorsalis, alcoholism, or spinal disease.
• Detrusor hyperactivity with impaired contractility (DHIC): High postvoid residual without outlet obstruction, common in frail older people.
• Functional: Inability or unwillingness to toilet because of physical, cognitive, psychological, or environmental factors.
• Other (rare): Bladder-sphincter dyssynergia, fistulas, reduced detrusor compliance; chronic urinary tract infection is not a common cause of UI.

Risk factors: Age-related changes, detrusor overactivity and uninhibited contractions, BPH, nocturia, atrophic urethritis, increased postvoid residual; decreased bladder capacity, dementia, depression, stroke, CHF, fecal incontinence, constipation, obesity, COPD, chronic cough, impaired ADL, Parkinson's disease.

Evaluation
- History: Precipitant urgency suggests detrusor overactivity; loss with cough, laugh, bend suggests stress; continuous leakage suggests intrinsic sphincter insufficiency or overflow. Onset, frequency, volume, timing, and precipitants (eg, caffeine, diuretics, alcohol, cough, medications) should be ascertained.
- Physical: Examine for orthostatic BP, heart rate, mental status examination, functional status impairment (eg, mobility, dexterity), volume overload, edema; bladder distension, rectal mass or impaction; cervical cord compression (interosseus muscle wasting, Hoffmann's or Babinski's signs); sacral root integrity (anal sphincter tone, anal wink, bulbocavernosus reflex, and perineal sensation).
  - Male GU: Prostate consistency, symmetry; for uncircumcised check phimosis, paraphimosis, balanitis.
  - Female GU: Atrophic vaginitis; pelvic support (see "Women's Health," p 111).

Testing
- Postvoid residual: If >100 mL repeat; still >100 mL suggests detrusor weakness, outlet obstruction or DHIC.
- Laboratory: Renal function tests, glucose, calcium, B_{12}; UA and urine C&S; urine cytology if hematuria or pain. PSA if cancer suspected.
- Voiding record: Record time and volume of incontinent/continent episodes, activities and time of sleep; knowing oral intake is sometimes helpful.
- Standing full bladder stress test: Relax perineum and cough once, immediate loss suggests stress; several seconds delay suggests detrusor overactivity.
- Urodynamic testing: Not routinely indicated; indicated before corrective surgery, when diagnosis is unclear, or when empiric therapy fails.
- Management: In a stepped approach, treat all transient causes first; avoid caffeine, alcohol, minimize evening intake of fluids.

Nonpharmacologic/Behavioral Therapy (First-Line Therapy)
- Detrusor instability: Timed toileting: shortest interval to keep dry; urge control: when urgency occurs, sit or stand quietly, focus on letting urge pass; when no longer urgent, walk slowly to the bathroom and void; when no incontinence for 2 days increase voiding interval by 30–60 minutes until voiding every 3–4 hours.
- Cognitively impaired persons: Prompted toileting (ask if patient needs to void) at 2- to 3-hour intervals while awake; encourage patients to report continence status, praise patient when continent and responds to toileting.
- Stress incontinence: Pelvic muscle (Kegel's) exercise. Isolate pelvic muscles (avoid thigh, rectal, buttocks contraction); sets of 10 contractions

Table 14. Drugs Used to Treat Urinary Incontinence

Types of Drugs	Mechanisms of Action	Types of Incontinence	Potential Adverse Effects	Specific Drugs and Dosages	Formulations
Anticholinergics/antispasmodics	↑ Bladder capacity; ↓ Involuntary contractions	Urge or mixed-urge; stress with detrusor overactivity	Dry mouth, blurry vision, ↑ intraocular pressure, delirium, constipation; *Imipramine only:* above effects plus postural ↓ blood pressure, cardiac conduction disturbances. May exhibit less dry mouth, depending on dosage	Oxybutynin (*Ditropan*): 2.5–5.0 mg BID-TID; Propantheline (*Pro-Banthine*): 15–30 mg TID (on empty stomach); Dicyclomine (*Bentyl*): 10–20 mg TID; Hyoscyamine (*Levsin*): 0.375–0.75 mg QID*; Tolterodine (*Detrol*): 1–2 mg BID; Imipramine (*Tofranil*): 10–50 mg qd	[Tablet 5, elixir 5 mg/5 mL] [7.5, 15]; [Tablet 10, 20, syrup 10 mg/5 mL]; [Tablet 125, elixir 125 mg/5 mL, sustained-release *Levsin* Timecaps .375–.75 po q12h .375 formulation] [1, 2]; [10, 25, 50]; [1, 2]
α-Adrenergic agonists	Increase urethral smooth muscle contraction	Stress with sphincter weakness	Headache, tachycardia, ↑ blood pressure; *Imipramine only:* see above	Pseudoephedrine (*Sudafed*): 15–30 mg TID (SR 120 mg qd BID); Phenylpropanolamine: 25 mg QID (SR 75 mg qd BID)	[Tablets 30, 60, elixir 30mg/5ml] [25, 50]
α-Adrenergic antagonists (See Chapter 30, Renal and Prostate Disorders)	Relax smooth muscle of urethra and prostate	Overflow or urge associated with BPH	Postural ↓ blood pressure, least with tamsulosin	Terazosin (*Hytrin*): 1–10 mg/day; Prazosin (*Minipress*): 1–2 mg TID*; Doxazosin (*Cardura*): 1–8 mg/day*; Tamsulosin (*Flomax*): 0.4–0.8 mg/day	[1, 2, 5, 10]; [1, 2.5]; [1, 2, 4, 8]; [Capsules 0.4]

* Extended-release and rapid-acting sublingual preparations available.

Source: Modified from Ouslauder JG. Urinary incontinence. In: Reuben DB, Yoshikawa TT, Besdine RW, eds. *Geriatrics Review Syllabus: A Core Curriculum in Geriatric Medicine* 3rd ed. Dubuque, Iowa: Kendall/Hunt Publishing Company for the American Geriatrics Society; 1996:131. Reprinted with permission.

at maximum strength 3–10 times/day, progressively longer (up to 10 seconds) contractions; follow-up and encouragement necessary.
- Pessaries may benefit women with vaginal or uterine prolapse.
- DHIC: Treat urge first; self-intermittent clean catheterization if needed.

Pharmacologic Therapy
Estrogen replacement may benefit both detrusor instability and stress incontinence; see p 111, "Women's Health," for recommended dose regimens. Other therapies are outlined in **Table 14,** p 27.

Catheter Care (use only for chronic urinary retention, nonhealing pressure ulcers in incontinent patients, and when requested by patients or families to promote comfort)
- Use closed drainage system only; avoid topical, or systemic antibiotics or catheters treated with antibiotics.
- Bacteriuria is universal; treat only if symptoms (ie, fever, inanition, anorexia, delirium), or if bacteriuria persists after catheter removal.
- Replace catheter if symptomatic bacteriuria then culture urine.
- Nursing facility patients with catheters should be kept in separate rooms.
- For acute retention catheterize for 7 days, then do voiding trial after catheter removal, never clamping.

Risk factors for catheter blockage: Alkaline urine, female gender, poor mobility, calciuria, proteinuria, copious mucin, proteus colonization, preexisting bladder stones.

Replacing catheters: For recurrent blockage change catheter every 7–10 days. Routine replacement not necessary unless monitoring is not adequate, in which case changing every 4–6 weeks is reasonable.

HEARING IMPAIRMENT

Definition
The most common sensory impairment in old age. To quantitate hearing ability, the necessary intensity (decibel = dB) and frequency (Hertz) of the perceived pure tone signal must be described.

Classification
Table 15 gives the hearing levels associated with varying degrees of hearing loss. Normal hearing threshold is 0–24 dB across all frequencies.
- Presbycusis: Characteristic old age hearing loss; most common cause of sensorineural loss; mainly high frequency loss and impaired speech discrimination and recruitment (an abnormal increase in sensation of loudness).
- Sensorineural hearing loss: Due to cochlear or retrocochlear pathology; both air and bone conduction thresholds are increased; causes: aging, eighth nerve damage from syphilis, viral meningitis, trauma, vascular events to eighth nerve or cortical tracts, acoustic neuroma, Meniere's disease.
- Conductive hearing loss: Occurs when sound transmission to inner ear is

impaired; bone conduction better than air conduction; external or middle ear disorders including otosclerosis; rheumatoid arthritis, Paget's disease.
- Central auditory processing disorders (CAPD): Loss of speech discrimination in excess of that from loss in hearing sensitivity; involves the CNS; seen in dementia and infrequently with presbycusis.

Evaluation

Screening: Note problems during conversation; ask about hearing dysfunction; HHIE-S is standardized questionnaire (see p 130); further screening can be done with a handheld audioscope or the whisper test—stand behind patient, 2 feet from the ear, cover the untested ear, fully exhale, whisper an easily answerable question. Refer patients who screen positive for audiologic evaluation.
- Audiometry: A pure tone audiogram documents the decibel loss across a range of frequencies, determines the pattern of loss (see "Classification"), and determines if loss is unilateral or bilateral. Speech reception is an important part of audiometry; if speech discrimination is less than 50% in patients with presbycusis, results with hearing aids may be poor.
- Aggravating factors: Sensorineural loss: medication ototoxicity (eg, aminoglycosides, loop diuretics, cisplatin), cerumen impaction. Conductive loss–cerumen impaction, external otitis.

Management
- Prevention: Avoid loud noise.
- Nonpharmacologic intervention:
  - Hearing aids are appropriate for most hearing-impaired persons; enhances select frequencies; should be individualized for each ear; both ears (binaural) amplification achieves best speech understanding; unilateral aid may be appropriate if asymmetrical speech discrimination or if hearing aid care is challenging.
  - Assistive listening devices place the microphone close to sound source and transmit to headphones or earpiece. Transmission is by wire or wireless (FM or infrared); some systems reduce signal-to-noise ratio which is useful for persons with CAPD.
  - Telephone device for the deaf (TDD): Receiver is a keyboard that allows the hearing impaired person to respond.
- Tips for communication with hearing-impaired: Stand 2–3 feet away, have the person's attention; have the person seated in front of a wall, which will help reflect sound; use lower-pitched voice; speak slowly and distinctly; rephrase rather than repeat; pause at the end of phrases or ideas.

Table 15. Degree of Hearing Loss and Recommended Step-Wise Interventions

Hearing Level (dB)	Degree of Loss	Treatment
25–40	Mild	Control background noise; louder speech
41–55	Moderate	Speak slowly and recommend hearing aid
56–70	Moderately severe	All of the above
71–89	Severe	All of the above
90	Profound	All of the above and behind the ear aid needed

VISUAL IMPAIRMENT

Definition
Visual acuity 20/40 or worse; severe visual impairment (legal blindness) 20/200 or worse.

Evaluation
Acuity testing: Near vision–Check each eye independently with glasses using handheld Rosenbaum card at 14" or Lighthouse Near Acuity Test at 16". Far vision–Snellen's wall chart at 10'. Visual fields: By confrontation formal Humphrey fields. Ophthalmoscopic evaluation. Tonometry using Tonopen.

Assessment
Causes of visual impairment in decreasing order of frequency:
- Refractive error
- Cataracts: Lens opacity on ophthalmoscopic examination. Risk factors: Age, sun exposure, smoking, steroids, diabetes.
- Age-related macular degeneration (ARMD): Atrophy of cells in the central macular region of retinal pigmented epithelium; on ophthalmoscopic examination white-yellow patches (drusen) or hemorrhage and scars in advanced stages. Risk factors: Age, sunlight exposure.
- Diabetic retinopathy: Microaneurysms, dot and blot hemorrhages on ophthalmoscopy with proliferative retinopathy ischemia and vitreous hemorrhage. Risk factors: Chronic hyperglycemia.
- Glaucoma: Intraocular pressure >21 mm mercury, optic cupping and nerve head atrophy, and loss of peripheral visual fields. Risk factors: Black race, age.

Management
- Prevention: Biennial full eye examinations for persons >65 years, annually for diabetic persons.
- Nonpharmacologic interventions: Cataract surgery (AHCPR guidelines) if acuity 20/50 or worse with symptoms of poor functional acuity; or if 20/40 or better with disabling glare or frequent exposure to low light situations, diplopia, disparity between eyes, or occupational need; or when cataract removal will treat another lens-induced disease (eg, glaucoma); or when cataract coexists with retinal disease requiring unrestricted monitoring (eg, diabetic retinopathy); ARMD photocoagulation for wet form. Glaucoma-surgical peripheral iridotomy or iridectomy or laser trabeculoplasty; used primarily when pressures poorly controlled by topical agents or when visual loss progresses. Diabetic retinopathy–laser treatment of proliferative retinopathy.
- Pharmacologic interventions: ARMD-zinc and antioxidants used but of questionable benefit. Diabetic retinopathy–glycemic control. Glaucoma: Some controversy, but therapy often indicated when pressures consistently elevated above 25 mm mercury (see **Table 16**, p 31).

Table 16. Agents for Treating Glaucoma

Drug	Strength	Dose	Metabolism	Caution/Side Effects
Sympathomimetics				
Epinephrine (*Epifrin, Glaucon*)	0.1%–2%	1 drop qd-bid	Liver	Hypertension, heart disease
Dipivefrin (*Propine*)	0.1%	1 drop bid	Eye, liver	Tachycardia, arrhythmia
Apraclonidine (*Iopidine*)	0.5, 1%	1–2 drops tid	Unknown	Caution in cardiovascular disease
β-Blockers				
Betaxolol (*Betoptic*)	0.25%–0.5%	1–2 drops bid	Liver	Hypotension, bradycardia
Carteolol (*Ocupress*)	1%	1 drop bid	Kidney	Bronchospasm
Levobunolol (*Betagan*)	0.25%–0.5%	1 drop bid	Liver	CNS symptoms, bradycardia
Metipranolol (*OptiPranolol*)	0.3%	1 drop bid	Liver	Heart failure
Timolol Gel (*Timoptic XE*)	0.25%–0.5%	1 drop bid-qd	Liver	Heart failure
Timolol Drops	0.25%–0.5%	1 drop bid	Liver	Heart failure
Miotics, Direct-Acting (not in narrow angle glaucoma)				
Pilocarpine (*Pilocar*)	0.25%–10%	1 drop qid	Tissues/ excreted in urine	Systemic cholinergic effects
Gel (*Pilopine HS*) (*Ocusert Pilo*)	4% 20–40 mg/hr	1/2" qhs Weekly	Tissues/ excreted in urine	Systemic cholinergic effects
Miotics, Cholinesterase Inhibitors (not in narrow angle glaucoma)				
Physostigmine	0.25%–0.5%	1–2 drops q 4–8 hours	Tissues/ excreted in urine	Cholinomimetic effects
Demecarium (*Humorsol*)	0.125%–0.25%	1–2 drops q 3 days-qd		Rhinitis, nausea
Echothiophate (*Phospholine Iodide*)	0.03%–0.25%	1 drop tid	Tissues	Bronchoconstriction, urinary
Isoflurophate (*Floropryl*)	0.025%	0.5 mg q 8–72 hr	Tissues	Frequency, CNS effects
Carbonic Anhydrase Inhibitors				
Dorzolamide (*Trusopt*)	2%	1 drop tid	Kidney	Not recommended in renal failure; sulfa allergy; hypokalemia; acidosis
Dichlorphenamide (*Daranide*)	50 mg	25–50 mg qd-tid	Liver/kidney	Not recommended in renal failure; sulfa allergy; hypokalemia; acidosis
Acetazolamide (*Diamox*)	125–500 mg	125–500 mg qd-qid	Kidney	Not recommended in renal failure; sulfa allergy; hypokalemia; acidosis
Methazolamide (*Neptazane*)	25–50 mg	50–100 mg bid-tid	Liver/kidney	Not recommended in renal failure; sulfa allergy; hypokalemia; acidosis
Other				
Latanoprost (*Xalatan*)	0.005%	1 drop qd	Liver/kidney	Change in iris color to brown
Brimonidine (*Alphagan*)	0.2%	1 drop bid	Liver	Low BP, fatigue, drowsiness, conjunctival blanching, lid reaction

- Low-vision rehabilitation/aids: Refer patients with uncompensated visual loss causing functional deficits. Aids include optical, nonoptical, low- and high-technology devices. Strategies include improved illumination, increased contrast, magnification, auditory and tactile feedback. Environmental modifications include using color contrast, floor lamps to reduce glare, motion sensors to turn on lights, high-technology options including video magnification with closed circuit television and word processing programs to enlarge text.
- Monitoring: Cataracts—periodic eye examinations; ARMD—use of Amsler's grid daily; glaucoma—tonometry every six months.

MALNUTRITION

Multidimensional Assessment
In the absence of valid nutrition screening instruments, clinicians may wish to probe for answers to the following questions:
- Does the patient's economic status pose a barrier to adequate nutritional intake?
- Is food of sufficiently high nutritional quality available to the patient?
- Are there dental problems that prohibit ingesting foods of high nutritional quality?
- Do the patient's medical illnesses interfere with the digestion or absorption of foods or cause additional nutritional requirements?
- Do limitations in the patient's functional capacity interfere with nutrition because of inability to shop, prepare meals, or feed him or herself?
- Do the patient's food preferences or cultural beliefs interfere with adequate nutritional intake?
- Does the patient have a good appetite?
- Does the patient have depressive symptoms?
- Because of the patient's other medical illnesses, does the patient have dietary restrictions (eg, low sodium diet) that interfere with adequate nutritional intake?

Anthropometrics: Weight on each visit and yearly height (see "Age-Related Physiologic Changes and Formulas," p 4).

Biochemical markers: Albumin (half-life, 18–20 days) can drop precipitously due to trauma, sepsis, or significant infection but may be valuable in nonacute settings; transferrin (half-life, 7 days); prealbumin (half-life, 48 hours) may be useful in monitoring nutritional recovery; low or falling values of serum cholesterol have prognostic value but may not be nutritionally mediated.

Management
Calculating basic energy (caloric) and fluid requirements:
- World Health Organization's energy estimates for adults over age 60 years:
  - Women (10.5) (weight in kg) + 596

– Men (13.5) (weight in kg) + 487
- Harris-Benedict energy requirement equations:
  – Women 655 + (9.6) (weight in kg) + (1.7) (height in cm) – (4.7) (age in years)
  – Men 66 + (13.7) (weight in kg) + (5.0) (height in cm) – (6.8) (age in years)

Depending on activity and physiologic stress levels, these basic requirements may need to be increased (eg, 25% for sedentary/mild, 50% for moderate, and 100% for intense/severe activity/stress). Fluid requirements for older persons without cardiac or renal disease are approximately 30 mL/kg of body weight per day.

Oral and enteral formulas: Many formulas are available (see **Table 17**, p 34); read the content labels and choose based on calories per mL, protein, fiber, lactose, and fluid load.

- Oral: Many (eg, Carnation Instant Breakfast, Health Shake) are milk-based and provide approximately 1.0–1.5 calories per mL.
- Enteral: Commercial preparations have between 0.5 and 2.0 calories per mL; most contain no milk (lactose) products. For patients who need fluid restriction, the higher concentrated formulas may be valuable but they may cause diarrhea. Because of reduced kidney function with aging, some recommend that protein should contribute no more than 20% of the formula's total calories. If formula is sole source of nutrition, consider formula that contains fiber (25 g/day is optimal).

Feeding Tube Management: Tips for Successful Tube Feeding
- Gastrostomy tube feeding may be either intermittent or continuous.
- Jejunostomy tube feedings must be continuous.
- Continuous tube feeding is associated with less frequent diarrhea but with higher rates of tube clogging.
- To prevent clogging and to provide additional free water, flushing with at least 30–60 cc of water 4 to 6 times a day is recommended. Sometimes carbonated beverages, cranberry juice, or meat tenderizer can restore patency to clogged tubes.
- Diarrhea, which occurs in 5% to 30% of persons receiving enteral feeding, may be related to the formula's lactose content (uncommon), the osmolality of the formula (uncommon), the rate of delivery, or other patient-related factors such as antibiotic use or impaired absorption.
- To help prevent aspiration, maintain a 30-degree elevation of the head of the bed during continuous feeding and for at least 2 hours following bolus feedings.

Parenteral Nutrition (PN) is indicated in those with digestive dysfunction precluding enteral feeding and delivers protein as amino acids, carbohydrate as dextrose, and fat as lipid emulsions.

- **Peripheral Parenteral Nutrition** (PPN) requires rotation of peripheral intravenous site every 72 hours. Solution osmolarity of less than 900 mOsm is recommended to reduce risk of phlebitis. (See **Table 18**, p 34.)
- **Total Parenteral Nutrition** (TPN) must be administered through a central catheter, which may be inserted peripherally (PICC).

Table 17. Examples of Lactose-Free Oral and Enteral Products

Product*	Kcal/mL	mOsm	Protein (g)	Water	Na (mEq)	K (mEq)
Oral–low residue						
Ensure	1.06	470	37.3	845	37	40
Ensure Plus	1.5	690	54.9	769	46	40
*Sustacal Basic**	1.06	650	37	850	37	41
Sustacal Plus	1.5	670	61	780	37	38
Oral–clear liquid						
Resource	1.06	430	33	842	24	1.3
Citrisource	0.76	700	37	876	10	1.6
Enteral–low residue						
Osmolite	1.06	300	37.2	841	28	26
Isocal	1.06	270	34	850	23	34
Enteral–low volume						
Deliver	2.00	640	75	710	35	43
Enteral–high fiber						
Ultracal	1.06	310	44	850	40	41
Jevity	1.06	310	44.4	830	40	40

* Also has "with fiber" product that is similar.

Table 18. Caloric Value and Osmolarity of Parenteral Solutions

Resolution	Caloric Value (Kcal/L)	Osmolarity (mOsm/L)
Dextrose (%)		
5	170	250
10	340	500
20	680	1000
60	1700	2500
70	2370	3500
Lipid emulsions (%)		
10	1100	230
20	2200	330–340

Source: Bçikston SJ. In: Ewald GA, McKenzie CR. *Manual of Medical Therapeutics.* 28th ed. Boston: Little, Brown and Company; 1995:36. Permission to reprint.

FALLS

Definition
An event that results in a person inadvertently coming to rest on the ground or lower level with or without loss of consciousness or injury. Excludes falls from major intrinsic event (stroke, syncope) or overwhelming environmental hazard.

Etiology
Typically multifactorial comprised of intrinsic (host) and external (environmental) and situation factors. A fall can be a common nonspecific sign for many acute illnesses in elderly individuals.

Evaluation

Rule out acute illness or underlying systemic/metabolic process (eg, infection, electrolyte imbalance as indicated by history or examination). For patient who has fallen:

– *History:* Determine circumstances of fall (eg, trip or slip, turning head); associated symptoms (eg, lightheadedness, chest pain); relevant comorbid conditions (eg, prior stroke, parkinsonism, cardiac disease); medication review, including OTC medications and alcohol use (see **Table 19,** below).

Table 19. Medications Associated With Increased Fall Risk	
Benzodiazepines	Laxatives
Other sedative-hypnotics	Skeletal muscle relaxants
Diuretics	Digoxin
Narcotics	Antiarrhythmics
Tricyclic antidepressants/SSRIs	Antihistamines
Antipsychotics	Vasodilators
Antihypertensives	MAOIs

SSRI = selective serotonin reuptake inhibitor; MAOI = monoamine oxidase inhibitor.

Table 20. Targeted Risk Factors and Corresponding Interventions	
Risk Factors	**Interventions**
Postural hypotension: drop in systolic blood pressure ≥20 mm Hg or to <90 mm Hg on standing	Behavioral recommendations, such as ankle pumps or hand clenching and elevation of head of bed; decrease in dosage, discontinuation, or substitution of medication that may contribute to hypotension. Pressure stockings (eg, Jobst); fludrocortisone (*Florinef*) .1 mg bid-tid [1] if indicated; midodrine (*Pro-Amatine*) 2.5-5.0 mg tid [2.5, 5].
Use of any benzodiazepine or other sedative-hypnotic agent	Education about the appropriate use of sedative-hypnotic agents; nonpharmacologic treatment of sleep problems, such as sleep restriction; tapering and discontinuation of medications.
Use of ≥ 4 prescription medications	Review of medications.
Environmental hazards for falls or tripping	Home safety assessment with appropriate changes, such as removal of hazards, safer furniture (correct height, more stable), installation of structures such as grab bars or handrails on stairs.
Any impairment in gait	Gait training; use of an appropriate assistive device; balance or strengthening exercises if indicated.
Any impairment in balance or transfer skills	Balance exercises, training in transfer skills if indicated; environmental alterations, such as grab bars or raised toilet seats.
Impairment in leg or arm muscle strength or range of motion (hip, ankle, knee, shoulder, hand, elbow)	Exercises with resistive bands and putty; resistance training 2-3x/week, increase resistance when able to complete 10 repetitions through the full range of motion.

Source: Modified from Tinetti ME, et al. A multifactorial intervention to reduce the risk of falling among elderly people living in the community. *N Engl J Med.* 1994;331:822. Permission to reprint.

- *Physical:* Assess for orthostatic BP, fever, hypothermia; head and neck, vision, or hearing impairment; heart arrhythmias, cardiac valve dysfunction; abnormal mental status, focal deficits, peripheral neuropathy, muscle weakness, instability, rigidity, tremor; musculoskeletal arthritic changes, motion limitations, podiatric problems, skeletal deformities.
- *Functional assessment:* Directly observe person's ability to get out of chair, observe gait and for ability to turn (see "Assessment Instruments," p 131), mobility, use of cane/walker/personal assistance, ambulation, activities of daily living (bathing, dressing, transfers).

Fall Prevention

Goal is to minimize risk of falling without compromising mobility and functional independence. Assessment for risk factors with targeted interventions to risk factors, such as impaired physical mobility, decreased vision and hearing, medication review, environmental modifications.

OSTEOPOROSIS

Commonly Used Definitions
- Established osteoporosis: occurrence of a minimal trauma fracture of any bone (World Health Organization [WHO]).
- Osteoporosis: low bone mass and microarchitectural deteriorations of bone tissue, leading to enhanced bone fragility and a consequent increase in fracture risk (NIH consensus conference).
- Osteoporosis: bone mineral density 2.5 standard deviations below that of younger normal individuals (WHO).

Evaluation
Some experts recommend excluding secondary causes (serum PTH, TSH, calcium, phosphorus, albumin, alkaline phosphatase, testosterone in men, renal and liver function tests, complete blood count). Less consensus on: Vitamin D levels, 24-hour urinary calcium, bone mineral density.

Toxins and Medications That Can Cause or Aggravate Osteoporosis
Tobacco, excessive alcohol, corticosteroids, heparin, some antiepileptic drugs (eg, phenytoin), possibly thyroxine (if over-replaced or suppressive doses).

Prevention
- Calcium (total intake of 1500 mg/day of elemental calcium if not given with estrogen or in men; 1000 mg if given with estrogen).
- Vitamin D, 400-800 IU/day.
- Weight-bearing physical activity and concurrent therapy to prevent falls, *and either*
- Estrogen (see p 113 for regimens) *or* raloxifene [*Evista*] 60 mg/day [60].
- Alendronate (*Fosamax*) 5 mg/day [5, 10, 40] (must be taken fasting with

water and patients must remain upright for at least 30 minutes after taking; relatively contraindicated in gastroesophageal reflux disease).

Treatment
- Calcium (total intake of 1500 mg/day of elemental calcium if not given with estrogen or in men; 1000 mg/day if given with estrogen).
- Vitamin D, 400-800 IU/day.
- Weight-bearing physical activity and concurrent therapy to prevent falls, *and one of the following*
- Estrogen (see p 113 for regimens) *or* raloxifene [*Evista*] 60 mg/day [60].
- Alendronate (*Fosamax*) 10 mg/day [5, 10, 40] (must be taken fasting with water and patients must remain upright for at least 30 minutes after taking; relatively contraindicated in gastroesophageal reflux disease), *or*
- Calcitonin (*Calcimar, Miacalcin*) 100 IU daily sc [200 IU/mL in 2-mL vials] or 200 IU (*Miacalcin*) [2-mL spray, 14 doses] (intranasally, alternate nostrils every other day). May also be helpful for analgesic effect in patients with acute vertebral fracture.

PRESSURE ULCERS

Definition
Any lesion caused by unrelieved pressure resulting in damage of underlying tissue; usually occurs over bony prominence.

Extrinsic Risk Factors
Pressure, shear, friction.

Intrinsic Risk Factors
Increased age, immobility (eg, stroke), malnutrition, sensory loss (eg, neuropathy), moisture (eg, incontinence), cognitive impairment.

Evaluation
Assessment of skin, especially for those with one or more risk factors. Determine severity of lesion using staging criteria:
- *Stage I:* Nonblanchable erythema of intact skin; heralds lesion of skin ulceration.
- *Stage II:* Partial-thickness skin loss involving epidermis and/or dermis; presents as abrasion, blister, or shallow crater.
- *Stage III:* Full-thickness skin loss involving damage or necrosis of subcutaneous tissue which may extend down to, but not through, underlying fascia; presents as deep crater with or without undermining of adjacent tissue.
- *Stage IV:* Full-thickness skin loss with extensive destruction, tissue necrosis or damage to muscle, bone, or supporting structures. May have associated undermining of sinus tracts.

Degree of damage is difficult to detect in darkly pigmented skin or presence of eschar. Failure of improvement over 2 weeks should result

in complete reassessment of risk factors and management strategies.
Heel ulcers: If no signs of infection or inflammation, do not debride dry eschar. If signs of infection or inflammation or wet eschar, should be surgically debrided; obtain vascular consult.

Management Goals, Prevention, and Treatment Strategies

Protect wound and surrounding skin from further trauma. Pressure reduction strategies: Frequent repositioning every 1–2 hours; pressure reducing/relieving cushions, mattresses. Avoid donut cushions. Reduce friction/shear: Head of bed < 30 degrees; use lift sheet; gentle removal of dressings.

Promote clean wound base/prevent infection. Moisture-retentive dressings, permeable to oxygen. Debridement if necrotic tissue/eschar present: Mechanical scissors, forceps, scalpel, wet-to-dry dressings; autolytic moisture-retentive dressings; chemical enzymes (see below). Cleanse as often as needed: Normal saline irrigations; absorb excess exudate: calcium alginates, absorbent powders, beads or pastes. Pack dead space: Packing strips; moistened saline gauze dressings.

Maintain moist wound environment. Moisture-retentive dressings: Transparent films, hydrogel, foams, calcium alginate, hydrocolloid.

Enhance systemic conditions. Provide nutritional support: Nutritional consultation, supplementation, hydration. Treat infections (odor, fever, erythema, increasing ulcer size): Removal of necrotic tissue and purulent drainage; systemic antibiotics for sepsis, osteomyelitis, spreading cellulitis. Topical antiseptics and antibiotics are generally not recommended.

Surgical repair. For deep-stage ulcers, may be only treatment of choice. Complete removal of surrounding tissue, scar, underlying bursa and bone. Large skin grafts or rotation flaps with thick subcutaneous fat or muscle are needed.

Wound Products: (Categorized by Type)

- *Hydrocolloids:* Comfeel, Cutinova Hydro, Restore, DuoDERM, Tegasorb, Hydrocol.
  - Wound use: Stages I and II (superficial stage III on very thin patients); purple, necrotic, sloughing wounds, light to moderate exudate. May be used with gels, alginates. Thin types of hydrocolloids reduce friction damage (eg, moving patients across bed linens).
  - Advantages: Comfortable, impermeable to external contaminants, supports autolytic debridement.
  - Disadvantages: NOT used for heavy exudate, infected wounds; nontransparent; edges can curl.
  - Hints: Characteristic odor and yellow exudate are normal with dressing removal. Be sure to have 1–1.5 inch margin around wound edge. "Border" types hold more securely. Contour dressing to increase adhesion and border cut edges with tape. Dressing changes vary 3–7 days to PRN.
- *Hydrogels:* Carrasyn, IntraSite, Normalgel, Curasol, HyFil, Woun'Dres, DuoDERM gel, Vigilon, NU-GEL.
  - Wound use: Partial and full thickness (stages II–IV); necrotic/sloughing; burns, radiation-damaged tissue.

Table 21. Wound and Pressure Ulcer Products by Drainage and by Pressure Ulcer Stage

Product	Light	Drainage Moderate	Heavy	Wound Stage I	II	III	IV	Color Purple	Black
Hydrocolloid	X	X		X	X			X	X
Hydrogel	X				X	X	X		X
Lubricating spray	X			X	X			X	X
Foam	X	X			X	X			
Nonadherent	X			X	X			X	
Transparent film	X			X	X			X	X
Calcium alginate		X	X			X	X		
Normal saline gauze		X	X			X	X		X
Enzymatic	X	X				X	X		X

- Advantages: Soothing-cooling; fills dead space; hydrates wounds, conforms to wounds; may use when infection present.
- Disadvantages: Requires secondary dressing; not for use of heavily exudating wounds. May macerate surrounding skin.
- Hints: Dressing frequency BID to QOD; use skin barrier (eg, No Sting, Skin Prep) to protect surrounding skin; use with N/S gauze to keep wound moist longer.
- *Exudate absorbers:* MeSalt, Calcium Alginates, KALTOSTAT, SORBSAN, Algasteril, Fibracol.
  - Wound use: Moderate to large amount of exudate; moist, sloughing wounds; wounds that require packing and absorption; infected exudating wounds.
  - Advantages: Absorbs up to 20x, fills dead space, easy to apply, maintains moist environment, less frequent changing than N/S gauze.
  - Disadvantages: Not for lightly exudating wounds; may dry wound bed.
  - Hints: May use gauze or transparent film dressing as secondary dressing. Dressing change frequency BID to 3 days.
- *Polyurethane foams:* Allevyn, LYOFOAM, PolyMOM, Ferris PolyMOM.
  - Wound use: Stage II–IV wounds with minimum to moderate exudate. Secondary dressing over packing and around drains.
  - Advantages: Nonadherent; conforms; use on infected wounds; some have attached surrounding adhesive to hold in place.
  - Disadvantages: Not for eschar; wounds with no exudate.
  - Hints: Skin sealant to protect intact surrounding skin. Dressing change frequency 1–5 days.
- *Lubricating spray:* Proderm, Granulex.
  - Wound use: Stage II wounds.
  - Advantages: Moisturizes; stimulates local circulation; easy to use; inexpensive; nonadhesive.
  - Disadvantages: Need to apply 2–3x/d; may stain.
  - Hints: Spray area and apply saturated secondary dressing.
- *Nonadherent dressings:* Adaptic, Telfa, Vaseline gauze, Xeroform.
  - Wound use: Donor sites; abrasions; skin tears; lacerations.

- Advantages: Nonadherent; readily available.
- Disadvantages: Limited moisture retention; needs secondary dressing to retain moisture, protect wound, and keep dressing in place.
- Hints: Dressing change frequency BID to QD.

- *Transparent adhesive dressings (TFD):* BIOCLUSIVE, OpSite, 3M, Tegaderm, Uniflex.
  - Wound use: Stage I and partial thickness Stage II. Lightly exudating; secondary dressing; some dry necrotic wounds.
  - Advantages: Impermeable to external contaminants; transparent; conformable; promotes autolytic debridement.
  - Disadvantages: Nonabsorbent; application can be difficult; not for infected wounds or fragile skin.
  - Hints: Protect surrounding skin with skin prep; shave surrounding hair; allow 0.5 inch around wound; dressing changes vary.

- *Gauze dressings:* Toppers; Kerlix.
  - Wound use: Wounds with exudate; dead space; tunneling; sinus tracts.
  - Advantages: Readily available; use with gels, NS; may use on infected wounds.
  - Disadvantages: Will disrupt wound healing if allowed to dry; needs secondary dressing.
  - Hints: Change q8 hours; pack wounds loosely; may macerate surrounding skin–protect with skin barrier.

- *Enzymatic debriding agents:* Santyl, Accuzyme, Rystan.
  - Wound use: Necrotic, sloughing wounds.
  - Advantages: Prepares wounds for surgical debridement; may be able to debride without surgery; works faster than gels/NS.
  - Disadvantages: Needs prescription; may cause burning sensation; works best in moist environment.
  - Hints: Crosshatch eschar to enhance enzyme activity; will not damage healthy tissue. With Santyl, company recommends use of polysporin powder first, then cover with Santyl.

- *Skin barriers:* Skin Prep, No Sting.
  - Use: Preparations used before application of adhesive materials.
  - Advantages: Protects skin when removing adhesive material; aids adhesion.
  - Hint: No Sting, alcohol free, doesn't hurt.

- *Moisture Barriers:* Vaseline, Proshield, Sooth and Cool, many other commercially available products.
  - Use: Protects skin from maceration due to frequent/heavy moisture; eg, urinary incontinence. May have zinc additive to promote drying and healing. Skin barrier pastes should only be used for severely incontinent patients.
  - Disadvantages: Skin barrier pastes can be difficult to remove from skin. Long-term use of barriers containing zinc can dry the skin.
  - Hints: Clean skin as often as necessary to reapply. Clean pastes off skin using mineral oil to avoid scrubbing skin. For severely moist and denuded skin, try sprinkling Stomahesive Powder first, dust off, and then apply moisture barrier treatment.

SLEEP DISORDERS

Classification
Insomnia (difficulty initiating or maintaining sleep), hypersomnolence, parasomnias (disorders of arousal, partial arousal, and sleep stage transition), and disturbance of the sleep-wake cycle, and sleep apnea.

Treatable Associated Medical/Psychiatric Conditions
Pain, paresthesias, cough, dyspnea from cardiac or pulmonary disease, gastroesophageal reflux, nocturia, depression, stress, anxiety, bereavement, adjustment disorders.

Medications That Cause or Aggravate Sleep Problems
Diuretics, caffeine, sympathomimetics including decongestants, bronchodilators, nicotine, alcohol, antidepressants, sedatives, levodopa, phenytoin, clonidine, beta-blockers, methyldopa, reserpine, quinidine, cortisone, progesterone.

Recommended Measures to Improve Sleep Hygiene
- Get out of bed at the same time each morning regardless of how much you slept the night before.
- Maintain a regular sleeping time, but don't go to bed unless sleepy.
- Decrease or eliminate naps, unless necessary part of sleeping schedule.
- Exercise daily, but not immediately before bedtime.
- Don't read or watch television in bed.
- Relax mentally before going to sleep; don't use bedtime as worry time.
- If hungry, have a light snack before bed (unless there are symptoms of gastroesophageal reflux or it is otherwise medically contraindicated), but avoid heavy meals at bedtime.
- Limit or eliminate alcohol, caffeine, and nicotine, especially before bedtime.
- Relax before bedtime, and maintain a routine period of preparation for bed (eg, washing up and going to the bathroom).
- Control the nighttime environment with comfortable temperature, quietness, and darkness.
- If it helps, use soothing noise, for example, a fan or other appliance or a "white noise" machine.
- Wear comfortable bedclothes.
- If unable to fall asleep within 30 minutes, get out of bed and perform soothing activity such as listening to soft music or reading (but avoid exposure to bright light during these times).
- Get adequate exposure to bright light during the day.

Principles of Prescribing Medications for Sleep Disorders
- Use lowest effective dose.
- Use intermittent dosing (2–4 times per week).
- Prescribe medications for short-term use (no more than 3–4 weeks).
- Discontinue medication gradually.
- Be alert for rebound insomnia following discontinuation.

41

Table 22. Useful Medications for Sleep Disorders in Elderly Persons

Drug	Class	Starting Dose	Usual Dose	Formulations	Half-life/ Metabolism/Excretion	Comments
Chloral hydrate (*Noctec*)	Nonbarbiturate, nonbenzodiazepine central nervous system depressant	500 mg (for hypnotic effect)	250–1000 mg (not to exceed 2 g as single dose or total daily dose)	[Capsule 250, 500; syrup 250, 500; suppository 324, 500, 648]	8 hours (active metabolite)/ K, L, L	Hypnotic effect lost after 2 weeks of continuous use Dyspepsia, flatulence, diarrhea Drug interactions (eg, decreased effect of phenytoin, transient increased effect of coumadin) Contraindicated in marked hepatic or renal impairment
Temazepam (*Restoril*)	Intermediate-acting benzodiazepine	7.5 mg	7.5–15 mg	[Capsules: 7.5, 15, 30]	8–10 hours (can be as long as 20–30 hours in elderly persons)/K	Daytime drowsiness may occur with repeated use Effective for sleep maintenance Delayed onset of effect
Estazolam (*ProSom*)	Intermediate-acting benzodiazepine	1 mg (healthy elderly persons) 0.4 mg (small or debilitated elderly persons)	0.5–1.0 mg	[Tablets: 1, 2]	12–18 hours/K	Rapidly absorbed, effective in initiating and maintaining sleep Slightly active metabolites that may accumulate
Zolpidem (*Ambien*)	Imidazopyridine (short-acting)	5 mg	5–10 mg	[Tablets: 5, 10]	1.5–4.5 hours (3 hours in elderly persons, 10 hours in those with hepatic cirrhosis)/L	Similar action to triazolam Reportedly little daytime carryover, tolerance, or rebound insomnia
Trazodone (*Desyrel*)	Sedating antidepressant (heterocyclic)	25–50 mg	25–100 mg	[Tablets: 50, 100, 150, 300]	12 hours/L	Moderate orthostatic effects Reportedly effective for insomnia with or without depression
Nefazodone (*Serzone*)	Sedating antidepressant	50 mg	50–100 mg	[Tablets: 100, 150, 100, 250]	2–4 hours/L	Antianxiety effect; less gastrointestinal upset and hypertension than with trazodone
Melatonin	Hormone	3 mg	3–6 mg	Various preparations		Not regulated by FDA

Source: Adapted from Alessi CA. Sleep Problems. In: Reuben DB, Yoshikawa TT, Bestine RW, eds. *Geriatrics Review Syllabus: A Core Curriculum in Geriatric Medicine,* 3rd ed. Dubuque, Iowa: Kendall/ Hunt Publishing Company for the American Geriatrics Society; 1996:174. Reprinted with permission.

Sleep Apnea

Definition: Repeated episodes of apnea or hypopnea during sleep with excessive daytime sleepiness or altered cardiopulmonary function.

Classification: Obstructive-airflow cessation as a result of upper airway closure in spite of adequate respiratory muscle effort; central-cessation of respiratory effort; mixed-features of obstructive and central.

Associated risk factors/clinical features: Family history, male gender, smoking, hypertension, obesity and increased neck circumference, snoring, upper airway structural abnormalities (eg, soft palate, tonsils).

Evaluation: Full night's sleep study (polysomnography) in sleep laboratory indicated for those who habitually snore and either report daytime sleepiness or have observed apnea; threshold for continuous positive airway pressure (CPAP) reimbursement by Medicare is 30 events/6-hr sleep or apnea-hypopnea index >5.

Nonpharmacologic treatment: Avoid use of alcohol or sedatives; weight loss in obese patients; sleeping in lateral rather than supine position; CPAP by nasal mask, nasal prongs, or mask that covers the nose and mouth (considered initial treatment for clinically important sleep apnea); oral appliances that keep the tongue in an anterior position during sleep or keep the mandible forward.

Pharmacologic therapy: Beneficial mostly in mild sleep apnea; protriptyline (*Vivactil*) 10–20 mg/day [5, 10] L (men frequently experience urinary hesitancy or frequency and impotence); fluoxetine (*Prozac*) 10–20 mg [10, 20, liquid 20 mg/5 mL] L.

Surgical therapy: Tracheostomy (indicated for patients with severe apnea who cannot tolerate positive pressure or other interventions are ineffective); uvulopalatopharyngoplasty (curative in fewer than 50% of cases); maxillofacial surgery (rare cases).

PAIN

Definition

An unpleasant sensory and emotional experience associated with actual or potential tissue damage.

Multidimensional Evaluation

Physical, functional, and psychological assessment. *Features in H & P:* May be less reliable in elderly because of memory impairment, depression, underreporting symptoms. Distinguish existing condition from new illness. *Pain assessment:* **PQRST P**rovocative (aggravating) and **P**alliative (relieving) factors; **Q**uality: Burning, stabbing, dull, throbbing; **R**egion (location); **S**everity: Scale of 0 (no pain) to 10 (worst can imagine); **T**iming when occurs. *Functional assessment:* Interference with activities: Sleep, eating, walking, rising/sitting, hygiene, sex, friends. *Psychological assessment:* Depression, anxiety, mental status (see "Assessment Instruments," p 126).

Pain Management

Initial Assessment: Distinguish acute from chronic pain.

- *Acute pain:* Distinct onset, obvious pathology, short duration.
- *Chronic pain:* Persistent >3 months, often associated with functional and psychological impairment, can fluctuate in character and intensity over time.
- *Common causes:* Arthritis, neuropathic or radiculopathic, cancer, leg cramps, claudication, postoperative, headaches.

First line for acute pain and short-term management: *Fixed* schedule of acetaminophen or opioids. Chronic pain: Multidisciplinary assessment and treatment; education for self-management and coping, combine drug and nondrug strategies. Anticipate and attend to depression and anxiety. Maximize function and quality of life.

ANALGESIC TREATMENT

WHO analgesic ladder

Step 1. Nonopioid drugs.

- Acetaminophen, up to 4 g/day;
- Nonsteroidal anti-inflammatory drugs (NSAIDs). Because of high toxicity in elderly people, NSAIDs (see **Table 34**, p 72) should be reserved for those with inflammatory conditions or in combination with an opioid for those with bone pain due to metastatic cancer. Avoid using large doses for a long period of time. Different toxicities, effectiveness for different patients. If one ineffective, try another.

Step 2. Low-dose opioid with nonopioid. Schedule 3 or 4 drugs (ie, no triplicate required). Dose limited by ceiling effects of the acetaminophen or NSAID, not the narcotic.

- Oxycodone (*Percocet, Percodan, Tylox*).
- Hydrocodone (*Vicodin, Lorcet*).

Step 3. Higher-dose opioid with nonopioid (see **Tables 23** and **24**, p 45 and p 46). Morphine is best understood and most predictable. Note: At some point all drugs will have ceiling effect (no additional benefit but additional side effects) (eg, codeine > 60 mg or hydrocodone/oxycodone > 10 mg).

Caveats for Elderly Individuals

- Avoid meperidine (*Demerol*) (metabolite produces CNS excitation), methadone or levorphanol (long half-life results in peak sedation days after pain is controlled), and fentanyl patch in opioid-naive patients. Fentanyl patch has long half-life in elderly, about 36 hours.
- For patients with severe pain, start with strong opioid.
- Patients with neuropathic pain can start with an adjuvant drug.
- Begin prophylactic laxative, osmotic, or stimulant. If taking fluids, increase fiber or psyllium. Titrate laxative dose up with opiate dose.
- Monitor for sedation, delirium, urinary retention, constipation, respiratory depression, and nausea.
- If considering long-term opioid treatment, evaluate not just pain management, but quality-of-life activities (eg, ability to attend social functions).
- Avoid starting 2 new drugs (adjuvant drug with opioid) simultaneously because it is difficult to distinguish side-effect profiles.
- Consider nonpharmacologic strategies for mild pain.

Other/Adjuvant Drugs
- Adjuvant drugs work best for neuropathic pain.
- May be only partially effective. Use with other medications.
- Adjuvant drugs can be toxic in elderly individuals.
- Antidepressants can be used to increase analgesia, particularly for neuropathic pain. (See **Table 25**, p 47.)
- Capsaicin is useful for a variety of neuropathic and arthritic pains.
- Anxiolytics (benzodiazepines, barbiturates) alone have no analgesic effect except for some neuropathic pain.

Nonpharmacologic Treatment
Combine nonpharmacologic with pharmacologic interventions.
- Cognitive therapy conducted by experienced professionals, distraction, imagery, hypnosis, biofeedback, relaxation techniques, music, coping skills.
- Repositioning, simple touch, massage, warmth.
- Exercise.
- Patient and caregiver education.
- Rehabilitation medicine consult (PT, OT): Mechanical devices to minimize pain and facilitate activity (eg, splints); transelectrical nerve stimulation (TENS); range-of-motion and ADL programs.
- Psychiatry pain management consult: For cognitive therapy recommendations; drug combinations (eg, adjuvant with opioid); withdrawal.
- Anesthesia pain consult for nerve blocks, neuroablation for neuropathic conditions not relieved by other treatments (postherpetic neuralgia, lumbar canal stenosis, neuropathy).

Table 23. Commonly Used Opioids in Elderly Individuals*

Drug (Trade Name[s])	Formulations (mg)	Indication/Comments
Codeine	[Tablets: 15, 30, 60; injection: 30, 60]	Mild-to-moderate pain
Hydromorphone (*Dilaudid, HydroStat*)	[Tablets: 1, 2, 3, 4, 8; injection: 1–4 mg/mL, 10 mg/mL; liquids: 5 mg/5 mL; suppository: 3 mg]	Moderate-to-severe pain
Morphine (*MSIR*) (*MS Contin, Oramorph SR*) (*MSIR*) (*Atramorph PF, Duramorph, Infumorph*) (*MSIR, Roxanol, OMS Concentrate, MS/L*) (*RMS, Roxanol, MS/S*)	[Tablets: 15, 30; controlled release: 15, 30, 60, 100, 200; soluble tabs: 10, 15, 30; injection: 0.5, 1–5, 8, 10, 15, 25, 50 mg/mL; solution: 10 mg/2.5 mL, 10 mg/ 5 mL, 20 mg/5 mL, 20 mg/mL, 100 mg/5 mL; suppository: 10, 20, 30]	Moderate-to-severe pain
Oxycodone (*Roxicodone*) (*Oxycontin*) (*Roxicodone*)	[Tablets: 5 mg; controlled release: 10, 20, 40; oral solution: 5 mg/mL]	Moderate-to-moderately severe pain
Oxymorphone (*Numorphan*)	[Injection: 1 mg/mL, 1.5 mg/mL; suppository: 5 mg]	Moderate-to-severe pain

*In elderly individuals, consider narcotic agonist analgesics: All are metabolized by liver and excreted primarily in urine. Renal/hepatic dysfunction may cause prolonged duration and cumulative effects. Similar side effects: Respiratory depression, nausea, hypotension, sedation. Avoid meperidine (*Demerol*) and propoxyphene (*Darvon*) in elderly individuals. Avoid agonist-antagonist: Pentazocine (*Talwin*), nalbuphine (*Nubain*) in elderly individuals.

Table 24. Approximate Equivalent Doses of Opioid Analgesics for Moderate-to-Severe Somatic and Visceral Pain

Drug (Trade Name[s])	Approximate Equianalgesic Oral Dose	Approximate Equianalgesic Parenteral Dose	Recommended Starting Dose >50 kg	Recommended Starting Dose <50 kg
Codeine	130 mg q3–4h	75 mg q3–4h	60 mg q3–4h (po) 60 mg q2h (IM/SQ)	1 mg/kg q3–4h (po)
Hydrocodone (in Lorcet, Lortab, Vicodin)	30 mg q3–4h	Not available	10 mg q3–4h (po)	0.2 mg/kg q3–4h (po)
Hydromorphone (Dilaudid)	7.5 mg q3–4h	1.5 mg q3–4h	6 mg q3–4h (po) 1.5 mg q3–4h (IM)	0.06 mg/kg q3–4h (po) 0.015 mg/kg q3–4h (IM)
Morphine*	30 mg q3–4h around-the-clock dosing 60 mg q3–4h single or intermittent dose	10 mg q3–4h	30 mg q3–4h (po) 10 mg q3–4h (IM/SQ)	0.3 mg/kg q3–4h (po) 0.1 mg/kg q3–4h (IM/SQ)
Oxycodone (Roxicodone, also in Percocet, Percodan, Tylox)	30 mg q3–4h	Not available	10 mg q3–4h (po)	0.2 mg/kg q3–4h (po)

*Source: Acute Pain Management Guideline Panel. Acute Pain Management: Operative or Medical Procedures and Trauma. Clinical Practice Guideline. AHCPR Pub. No. 92-0032. Rockville, MD: Agency for Health Care Policy and Research, Public Health Service, U.S. Department of Health and Human Services. Feb. 1992.

Table 25. Other/Adjuvant Drug Therapy for Pain Relief in Elderly Individuals

Class Drug [Trade Name(s)]	Pain Indication	Starting Dose	Formulations	Metabolized	Comments
Antidepressant					
Venlafaxine (*Effexor*)	Fibromyalgia Muscle Neuropathic	25 mg BID	[Tablets: 25, 37.5, 50, 75, 100]	L	Less anticholinergic effect and sedation than tricyclics
Nortriptyline (*Aventyl, Pamelor*)	Neuropathic Migraine Tension headaches Arthritic	10 mg qhs BID	[Capsules: 10, 25, 50, 75]	L	Less sedating and anticholinergic effects than other tricyclics
Doxepin (*Sinequan*)	Same as above	10 mg qhs BID	[Capsules: 10, 25, 50]	L	Sedating; start at hs.
Desipramine (*Norpramin, Pertofrane*)	Same as above	10 mg qhs BID	[Tablets: 10, 25, 50, 75, 100, 150; capsules: 25, 50]	L	Least sedating and anticholinergic effects of tricyclics
Anticonvulsants					
Gabapentin (*Neurontin*)	Neuropathic	100 mg BID	[Capsules: 100, 300, 400]	R	Start low, increase slowly—100 mg/d q5d. May cause drowsiness
Lamotrigine (*Lamictal*)	Neuropathic	25 mg BID	[Tablets: 25, 100, 150, 200]	R	Rash common, dizziness, nausea, CNS effects
Carbamazepine (*Tegretol*)	Neuropathic	100 mg BID	[Tablets: 200; chewable tablets: 100; suspension: 100 mg/5 mL]	L	May cause agitation, confusion in elderly, dizziness, drowsiness, many drug interactions; helpful when withdrawing opioid
Other					
Capsaicin (*Zostrix, Capzasin, R-Gel, Capsin, No pin-HP*)	Arthritic Neuralgias	3–4 x/day	[Creams, lotion, gel, roll-on: 0.025%, 0.075%]	—	Renders skin and joints insensitive by depleting and preventing reaccumulation of substance P in peripheral sensory neurons; may cause burning sensation; instruct patient to wash hands after application to prevent eye contact; do not apply to open or broken skin

47

DEPRESSION

Evaluation/Assessment

Recognizing and diagnosing late-life depression can be difficult. Older patients may complain of lack of energy, or their symptoms may be attributed to old age or other medical conditions. Often, these complaints will not be mentioned to a health care professional.

Medical Evaluation

Thyroid function – TSH; serum chemistries and electrolytes; urinalysis; CBC.

DSM-IV Criteria for Major Depressive Episode (abbreviated)

Five or more of the following symptoms have been present during the same 2-week period and represent a change from previous functioning; at least one of the symptoms is either (1) depressed mood or (2) loss of interest or pleasure.

- Depressed mood;
- Loss of interest or pleasure in activities most of the day;
- Significant weight loss or gain (not intentional), or decrease or increase in appetite;
- Insomnia or hypersomnia;
- Psychomotor agitation or retardation;
- Fatigue or loss of energy;
- Feelings of worthlessness or excessive or inappropriate guilt;
- Diminished ability to think or concentrate, or indecisiveness;
- Recurrent thoughts of death, recurrent suicidal ideation, suicidal attempt or plan.

The *DSM-IV* criteria are not specific for the older adult; however, it is recognized that cognitive symptoms in the older adult may be more prominent. The Geriatric Depression Scale is a useful instrument for screening and diagnosing depression (see "Assessment Instruments," p 129).

Management

Treatment should be individualized based on history and severity of illness as well as concurrent illnesses. Treatments may be used individually or in combinations.

- **Nonpharmacologic:** For mild to moderate depression or in combination with pharmacotherapy; cognitive-behavioral therapy; interpersonal therapy; psychodynamic psychotherapies.
- **Pharmacologic:** For mild, moderate or severe depression. With the exception of psychostimulants, the duration of therapy should be at least 6 months following remission for patients experiencing their first depressive episode. Patients with a history of previous episodes of major depression should be treated a minimum of 12 months following remission and some may require indefinite antidepressant therapy.
  - **Other Antidepressants** - Trazodone (*Desyrel*): dose 75-150 mg/day, sedation may limit dose; [Tablet 50, 100, 150, 300 mg]; L.

Table 26. Preferred Antidepressants for Older Adults

Generic Name (Brand) Strength and Formulation	Initial Dose	Usual Dose	Elimination	Situations Favoring Use/Comments
Tricyclic Antidepressants				
Nortriptyline (*Aventyl*) [Capsule: 10, 25, 50, 75; solution: 10 mg/5mL]	10–25 mg qhs	75–150 mg/day	L	Past response, melancholia Therapeutic window (serum level) 50-150 ng/mL; baseline EKG.
Desipramine (*Norpramin*) [Capsule: 25, 50 mg; tablets: 10, 25, 50, 75, 100, 150 mg]	10–25 mg qhs	50–150 mg/day	L	Past response, melancholia Therapeutic serum level >115 ng/mL; baseline EKG; may be stimulating
Selective Serotonin Reuptake Inhibitors				
Paroxetine (*Paxil*) [Tablets: 10, 20, 30, 40 mg]	10–20 mg qam or qpm	20–30 mg/day	L	Mild-moderate depression, heart disease, BPH, glaucoma; lower anticholinergic effects than the TCA, relieves irritability, no EKG
Sertraline (*Zoloft*) [Tablets: 25, 50, 100 mg]	25 mg qam	50–100 mg/day	L	See paroxetine; less anticholinergic and sedating than paroxetine
Other				
Bupropion (*Wellbutrin*) [Tablets: 75, 100 mg; tablets: SR 100, 150 mg]	25–50 mg bid (SR) or tid	50 mg tid	L	Poor response to TCA or SSRI Safe in CHF, may be stimulating; can lower seizure threshold
Alternative Agents (in no particular order of preference)				
Mirtazapine (*Remeron*) [Tablets: 15, 30 mg]	7.5 mg qhs	15–45 mg/day	L	May increase appetite
Nefazodone (*Serzone*) [Tablets: 100, 150, 200, 250 mg]	50 mg bid	200–400 mg/day	L	Useful when anxiety is present; does not negatively affect sleep
Venlafaxine (*Effexor*) [Tablets: 25, 37.5, 50, 75, 100 mg]	25–50 mg bid	37.5–225 mg/day	L	Low anticholinergic activity, minimal sedation and hypotension
Methylphenidate (*Ritalin*) [Tablets: 5, 10, 20 mg]	2.5–5 mg at 7 AM and noon	5–10 mg at 7 AM and noon	L	Role in the treatment of depression in the medically ill elderly; response usually in 3-4 days; may use as an adjunct for moderate to severe depression

- **Tricyclic antidepressants:** Amitriptyline (*Elavil*): dose: 10-25 mg/day; avoid in elderly patients; [Tablet 10, 25, 50, 75, 100, 150 mg; Injection 10 mg/mL (10 mL)]; L. amoxapine (*Asendin*): dose: 50-150 mg/day; avoid in elderly patients; [Tablet 25, 50, 100, 150 mg]; L. clomipramine (*Anafranil*): dose: 100-250 mg/day; not used as antidepressant for elderly patients; [Capsule 25, 50, 75 mg]; L. doxepin (*Sinequan, Adepin*): dose: 25-150 mg/day; best to avoid in elderly patients; [Capsule 10, 25, 50, 75, 100, 150 mg; concentrate, oral, 10 mg/mL (120 mL)]; L. imipramine (*Tofranil*):

dose 50-150 mg/day; avoid as an antidepressant in elderly patients; [Capsule, as pamoate: 75, 100, 125, 150 mg; Injection 12.5 mg/mL (2 mL); Tablet, as hydrochloride: 10, 25, 50 mg]; L. protriptyline (*Vivactil*): dose: 15-20 mg/day; avoid as an antidepressant in elderly patients; [Tablet 5, 10 mg]; L. trimipramine: (*Surmontil*): dose 25-100 mg/day; avoid as an antidepressant in elderly patients; [Capsule 25, 50, 100 mg]. L.

- **Selective serotonin reuptake inhibitors (SSRIs):** Fluoxetine (*Prozac*): dose: 10-20 mg qam; [Capsule 10, 20 mg; Liquid 20 mg/5 mL]; L. fluvoxamine (*Luvox*): dose: 100-300 mg/day, given bid; [Tablet 50, 100 mg]; L.

- **Monoamine oxidase inhibitors (MAOIs):** Phenelzine (*Nardil*): dose: 15-60 mg/day, tid-qid; [Tablet 15 mg]; L & K. Tranylcypromine (*Parnate*): dose: 20-40 mg/day, bid; [Tablet 10 mg]; K.

- **Psychostimulants:** Dextroamphetamine (*Dexedrine*): dose: 5-10 mg at 7 AM and noon: [Tablet 5 mg, 10 mg; Elixir 5 mg/5 mL]; L & K.

– **Electroconvulsive Therapy (ECT):** Generally safe and very effective. Indications: Severe depression when a rapid onset of response is necessary, depression resistant to drug therapy, patients who are unable to tolerate antidepressants, previous response to ECT, psychotic depression, severe catatonia, or depression with Parkinson's disease. Complications: Confusion, falls, memory loss, arrhythmias, bronchospasm, aspiration. Contraindications: Increased intracranial pressure, intracranial tumor, myocardial infarction within 3 months (relative) or stroke within 1 month (relative).

ANXIETY

Anxiety disorders are less prevalent in elderly individuals than in younger adults. New-onset anxiety in the elderly is usually secondary to medical illness, depression, medication side effects or withdrawal from drugs.

DSM-IV recognizes a variety of anxiety disorders including
- Panic disorder, with or without agoraphobia.
- Agoraphobia without a history of panic.
- Social phobia.
- Specific phobia.
- Generalized anxiety disorder (GAD).
- Obsessive-compulsive disorder (OCD).
- Acute stress disorder.
- Posttraumatic stress disorder.
- Anxiety disorder due to a general medical condition and substance-induced anxiety disorder.

The latter condition and GAD are the most common anxiety disorders occurring in older persons.

Differential Diagnosis/Evaluation

- Medical conditions
  - Cardiovascular – Arrhythmias, angina, myocardial infarction, CHF.
  - Respiratory – COPD, asthma, pulmonary embolism.
  - Endocrine – Hyperthyroidism, hypoglycemia, pheochromocytoma.
  - Neurologic – Movement disorders, temporal lobe epilepsy.
- Medications
  - Sympathomimetics – Pseudoephedrine.
  - Thyroid hormones – Overreplacement.
  - Psychotropics – Antidepressants (eg, SSRIs; neuroleptics; stimulants).
  - Steroids.
  - Caffeine.
  - Nicotine.
- Withdrawal states
  - Alcohol.
  - Sedatives, hypnotics, benzodiazepines.
- Depression.

Evaluation of Anxiety

- History of present illness.
- Past psychiatric history.
- Drug review – Prescribed, OTC, alcohol.
- Mental status evaluation – Looking for signs/symptoms of anxiety.
- Physical examination – Focus on signs and symptoms of anxiety (eg, tachycardia, hyperpnea, sweating, tremor).
- Consider anxiety rating scale (eg, Hamilton Anxiety Scale or Beck Anxiety Inventory).
- Laboratory tests – CBC, blood glucose, thyroid function tests, B_{12} and folate, ECG, drug/alcohol screening, if warranted.

Nonpharmacologic Management

Cognitive-behavior therapy (CBT) may be useful for GAD, panic disorder, and OCD. May be effective alone in less severe cases but mostly used in conjunction with pharmacotherapy. CBT requires a motivated patient who is cognitively intact.

Pharmacologic Management

A variety of compounds have been used as anxiolytics: Benzodiazepines, buspirone, antidepressants, neuroleptics, beta-blockers, and antihistamines.

Benzodiazepines

- Best studied, most utilized for acute anxiety, GAD, panic, OCD.
- Short half-life drugs such as: oxazepam (*Serax*): dose 10–15 mg bid-tid [10, 15, 30], alprazolam (*Xanax*): dose 0.125–0.25 mg bid initially [0.25, 0.5, 1, 2], lorazepam (*Ativan*): dose 0.5–2 mg in 2 to 3 divided doses [0.5, 1, 2] preferred. These are inactivated by direct conjugation in liver and therefore not affected by aging.
- Long-acting benzodiazepines (eg, flurazepam, diazepam, chlordiazepoxide) are linked to cognitive impairment, falls, sedation, psychomotor impairment.

- Dependence, tolerance, withdrawal are problems, more so with short-acting benzodiazepines.
- Potentially fatal if combined with alcohol or other CNS depressants.
- Only short-term (60–90 days) use is recommended.

Buspirone
- Serotonin 1A partial agonist effective in GAD and anxiety symptoms accompanying general medical illness.
- Not effective for acute anxiety, panic, or OCD.
- May take 2–4 weeks for optimal effect.
- Recommended geriatric dose: 15–20 mg bid [5, 10, 15, 30].
- No dependence, tolerance, withdrawal, CNS depression or significant drug-drug interactions.

Table 27. Summary of Management of Anxiety Disorders

Anxiety Disorder	Primary Treatment	Alternative Treatment
GAD	Buspirone, benzodiazepines	CBT
Panic disorder	SSRI antidepressants	CBT, alprazolam, imipramine
OCD	SSRIs	CBT, clomipramine

Source: Adapted from: Sheikh JI. Anxiety disorders. In: Coffee CE, Cummings JL, eds. *Textbook of Geriatric Neuropsychiatry*. Washington, DC: APA Press; 1994:279–296. Reprinted with permission.

PSYCHOTIC DISORDERS

Differential diagnosis of psychotic symptoms in the elderly includes:
- Schizophrenia (early onset, before age 45 versus late onset).
- Major depression with psychotic features.
- Bipolar affective disorder with psychosis.
- Delirium with psychosis.
- Dementia with psychosis.
- Late-life delusional (paranoid) disorder.
- Drug-related causes, eg, antiparkinsonian agents, anticholinergics, benzodiazepines (including withdrawal); alcohol (including withdrawal), stimulants, steroids, cardiac drugs, ie, digitalis.
- Medical disorders: Hypo- or hyperglycemia, hypo- or hyperthyroidism, sodium/potassium imbalance, Cushing's syndrome, Parkinson's disease, B_{12} and folate deficiency, sleep deprivation, AIDS.
- Structural brain lesions – tumor or stroke.
- Seizure disorder (eg, temporal).

Risk Factors for Psychotic Symptoms in Elderly
- Cognitive impairment – acute or chronic progressive.
- Sensory impairment.
- Female gender.
- Social isolation.
- Bedfast status.

Table 28. Representative Neuroleptics

Drug Class	Representative Agents	Side Effects (Metabolism)	Geriatric Dosage Range (Total mg/day; frequency/day)	Formulations Available	Metabolism/Excretion
Low potency	Chlorpromazine (*Thorazine*)	Sedation Orthostasis Anticholinergic Tardive dyskinesia	25–200 (1–3)	[Scored tablet 10, 25, 50, 100, 200, syrup 10 mg/5 mL]	L, K
	Thioridazine (*Mellaril*)			[Tablets 10, 15, 25, 50, 100, 150, 200, suspension 25, 100 mg/5 mL]	L, K
Intermediate potency	Loxapine (*Loxitane*)	Anticholinergic Orthostasis Sedation Tardive dyskinesia	2.5–20 (1–3)	[Tablets 5, 10, 25, 50, liquid 25 mg/mL]	L, K
High potency	Haloperidol (*Haldol*)	EPS Tardive dyskinesia	0.5–2 (1–3)	[Tablets 5, 1, 2, 5, 10, 20, liquid 2 mg/mL, depot 100–200 mg IM q4 wk]	L, K
Novel agents	Clozapine (*Clozaril*)	Sedation Agranulocytosis Orthostasis Anticholinergic Weight gain	25–150 (1)	[Tablets 25, 100 mg]	L
	Risperidone (*Risperdal*)	Orthostasis EPS at high doses	0.5–2 (1–2)	[Scored tablets 1, 2, 3, 4 mg, liquid 100 mL 1 mg/mL]	L, K
	Olanzapine (*Zyprexa*)	Sedation Anticholinergic EPS at high doses Weight gain	2.5–10 (1)	[Tablets 5, 10 mg]	L
	Quetiapine (*Seroquel*)	Sedation Cataracts Nasal stuffiness Orthostasis	25–50 (1–2)	[Tablets 25, 50 mg]	L, K

53

Treatment of Psychotic Symptoms

Nonpharmacologic: If symptoms are secondary to toxic, organic, or underlying medical causes – alleviation of these factors is paramount. Identifiable psychosocial triggers should be addressed. Delirium with psychotic features should resolve once the etiology of the delirium is determined.

Pharmacologic: If psychotic symptoms are severe or frightening or affect the potential safety of the patient or others – neuroleptic therapy is warranted. Remember that neuroleptics may cause akathisia.

Table 29. Management of Side Effects of Neuroleptics		
Side Effect	**Treatment**	**Comment**
Drug-induced Parkinsonism	Lower dose or switch to novel neuroleptic	Often dose related; increase in elderly with traditional neuroleptics
Akathisia	Decrease dosage, beta-blocker (eg, propranolol 20–40 mg/day) or switch to novel neuroleptic	Also seen with olanzapine and risperidone
Hypotension	Slow titration; reduce dose; change drug class	Most common with low-potency neuroleptics
Sedation	Reduce dose; give at bedtime; change drug class	Most common with low-potency neuroleptics
Tardive dyskinesia	Stop drug (if possible); change to novel neuroleptic	Increased risk in elderly; may be irreversible

Periodic (5–6 months) reevaluation of neuroleptic dose and ongoing need is important. (See OBRA Regulations, p 137.) Older persons are particularly sensitive to side effects of neuroleptics. They are also at higher risk of developing tardive dyskinesia (TD). Periodic use of a side-effect scale such as the AIMS (see "Assessment Instruments," p 126) is highly recommended.

ALCOHOL AND DRUG ABUSE

Definition

- Possible alcohol dependence: *Diagnostic and Statistical Manual of Mental Disorders-IV* (*DSM-IV*). Three or more of the following:
  Tolerance, or requiring more alcohol to get "high"; withdrawal, or drinking to relieve/prevent withdrawal; drinking in larger amounts, or for a longer period of time than intended; persistent desire to drink, or unsuccessful efforts to cut down or control drinking; a lot of time spent in activities necessary to obtain or use alcohol or recover from effects; important occupational, social, or recreational activities given up or reduced because of drinking alcohol; drinking continues despite knowledge of persistent/recurrent physical or psychological problems likely to be caused/worsened by alcohol.
- Possible alcohol abuse: (*DSM-IV*). One or more of the following:
  Recurrent drinking resulting in the failure to fulfill major obligations at work or in the home; recurrent drinking in situations where it is physically hazardous; recurrent alcohol-related legal problems; continued drinking

despite persistent or recurrent social problems caused or worsened
by alcohol.
- Harmful drinking (2-3 drinks/day): increased risk of hypertension; increased
  risk of some cancers (eg, head and neck, and breast in women). Possible
  increased risk for hip fracture and other injury.
- Drug abuse: Illicit drug use is uncommon in old age; prescription
  drug abuse is probably more common. Drugs most often implicated:
  benzodiazepines, sedative-hypnotics, opioid analgesics, stimulants,
  and barbiturates.

Evaluation
- Alcohol misuse screening: CAGE questionnaire has been validated in the
  older population. Have you ever felt you should **C**ut down? Does others'
  criticism of your drinking **A**nnoy you? Have you ever felt **G**uilty about
  drinking? Have you ever had an "**E**ye opener" to steady your nerves or get
  rid of a hangover? Positive response to any suggests problem drinking.
- Detecting harmful drinking: May be missed by CAGE; ask quantity and
  frequency: How many drinks per week? How many drinks on those days?
  Maximum intake on any one day? What type (ie, beer, wine, or liquor)?
  What is in "a drink"?

Aggravating Factors
- Alcohol dependence or abuse: Often missed in old age because of
  reduced social and occupational functioning; signs more often are poor
  self-care, malnutrition. The Michigan Alcoholism Screening Test
  (MAST-G) (see "Assessment Instruments," p 136) probes these issues.
- Alcohol and aging: Higher blood levels per amount consumed due to
  decreased lean body mass and total body water; concomitant medications
  may interact with alcohol.
- Prescription drug abuse: Unrecognized/untreated depression and anxiety,
  chronic pain, sleep problems.

Management
- Alcohol guidelines: No more than one drink/day after age 65; one drink/day
  probably reduces cardiovascular risk.
- Psychosocial interventions: Problem drinking/alcohol misuse. Brief intervention – Educate patient on effects of current drinking, point out current
  adverse effects.
- Alcohol dependence/abuse: Self-help groups (ie, Alcoholics Anonymous);
  professional (ie, psychodynamic, cognitive-behavioral, counseling, social
  support, family therapy, age-specific inpatient/outpatient).
- Pharmacologic interventions for alcoholism: Disulfiram (*Antabuse*)—
  125-500 mg po qd; [250, 500 mg, scored tablet] not effective in clinical trials;
  serious cardiovascular side effects. Naltrexone (*ReVia*)—25 mg po qd x
  2 days then 50 mg po qd; [50 mg, scored tablet] metabolize liver/kidney;
  monitor liver enzymes; useful as adjunct to psychosocial therapy;
  contraindicated in renal failure.
- Acute alcohol withdrawal (see "Delirium," p 18).

CARDIOVASCULAR DISEASE

ACUTE MYOCARDIAL INFARCTION (MI) MANAGEMENT

Evaluation/Assessment

- As in younger persons, diagnosis is made by cardiac enzyme rises, with or without ECG changes.
- Presentation frequently atypical—suspect MI with atypical chest pain; arm, jaw, or abdominal pain (with or without nausea); acute functional decline.
- Risk factors for acute MI in older adults. *Strong:* Previous MI or angina, age, hypertension, smoking, diabetes. *Weak:* Dyslipidemia (except in those with overt coronary disease), obesity, family history, sedentary lifestyle.

Management

Thrombolytic therapy for Q-wave MI (chest pain <12 hrs, ≥1 mm ST-segment elevation).

- Age is not a contraindication.
- Absolute contraindications: Active internal bleeding; history of cerebral hemorrhage; pericarditis; aortic dissection; cerebral aneurysm, arteriovenous malformation, or neoplasm; allergy to thrombolytics.
- Relative contraindications: Recent (within 10 days) trauma, major surgery, or head injury; GI/GU bleeding or stroke within 6 months; prolonged (>10 minutes) CPR; chronic liver disease; systolic BP >200; diastolic BP >110; stroke with residual deficit; arterial puncture or dental extraction within 2 weeks; proliferative diabetic retinopathy; prior (<1 year) thrombolytic therapy.

Percutaneous transluminal coronary angioplasty (PTCA) or emergent coronary artery bypass grafting (CABG) are alternatives to thrombolytic therapy.

Pharmacologic Management. For both Q- and non–Q-wave MI:

- *Aspirin*, at least 81 mg qd, should be started at the time of MI and continued indefinitely.
- *Heparin* should be given acutely. For patients undergoing thrombolytic therapy or immediate PTCA, those with continuing pain or those with indications for warfarin therapy (see below), give 5,000 units bolus IV + 1,000 units/hr IV; check activated partial thromboplastin time q6h (target 1.5–2.0 X control). Otherwise, give 7,500 units sq q12h until patient is fully ambulatory. *Warfarin* therapy is indicated in post-MI patients with atrial fibrillation, left ventricular thrombosis, or large anterior infarction (target INR 2.0–3.0).
- *β-Blockers* should be given acutely and continued chronically unless systolic failure or pronounced bradycardia is present. Acute phase: Atenolol (*Tenormin*), 5 mg IV over 5 minutes and repeat in 10 minutes; or metoprolol (*Lopressor*) 5 mg IV 95 minutes up to a total of 15 mg. Begin chronic phase within 1-2 hours: Atenolol 25–100 mg po qd or metoprolol, 50–200 mg po bid.

56

- *Nitroglycerin* is indicated acutely for persistent ischemia, hypertension, or CHF. Begin at 5–10 µg/min IV and titrate to pain relief, SBP >90, or resolution of ECG abnormalities.
- *Oxygen:* 2–4 L/min via nasal cannula should be given acutely.
- *Angiotensin-converting enzyme inhibitors* (ACEI) should be started approximately 3 days following an MI in cases with systolic dysfunction. Examples: Captopril (*Capoten*), 6.25–25 mg po bid/tid; enalapril (*Vasotec*), 2.5–20 mg po qd/bid; lisinopril (*Prinivil, Zestril*), 2.5–20 mg po qd.
- *Calcium channel blockers* should be used cautiously, only in non–Q-wave infarctions without systolic dysfunction and a contraindication to β-blockers.
- Lipid-lowering therapy (see p 58) to achieve target levels (total cholesterol <160 mg/dL, LDL cholesterol <100 mg/dL, HDL cholesterol >45 mg/dL) should be initiated by the time of hospital discharge.
- At time of discharge, prescribe rapid acting nitrates prn. Sublingual nitroglycerin (eg, *Nitrostat*) 0.2–0.6 mg [0.15, 0.3, 0.4, 0.6] every 5 minutes for maximum of 3 doses in 15 minutes; sublingual isosorbide dinitrate (*Isordil, Sorbitrate*) 2.5–5 mg [2.5, 5, 10]; nitroglycerin spray (*Nitrolingual*) [0.4 mg/spray] 1–2 oral sprays under tongue, every 5 minutes for maximum of 3 doses in 15 minutes.
- Longer acting nitrates if symptomatic angina and treatment will be medical rather than surgical or angioplasty. May be combined with beta blockers and/or calcium channel blockers. Isosorbide dinitrate (*Isordil, Sorbitrate*): 10–40 mg po 3 times daily 6h apart [Tab: 5, 10, 20, 30, 40; chew tab: 5, 10]; SL tabs: 1 prn [2.5, 5, 10]; Sustained release (*Isordil Tembids, Diltrate* SR): 40–80 po bid/tid [40]. Isosorbide mononitrate (*ISMO, Monoket*): 20 mg po twice daily with doses 7h apart [10, 20]; Extended release (*Imdur*): Start 30–60 po qd, maximum 240 mg/day [30, 60, 120]. Nitroglycerin ointment 2% (*Nitro-Bid, Nitrol*): start 0.5 inch q8h, maintenance 1-2 inches q8h, maximum 4-5 inches q4 h [15mg/inch]. Nitroglycerin sustained release (*Nitro-Bid*) start 2.5 po bid/tid, then titrate upward as needed [2.5, 6.5, 9]. Nitroglycerin transdermal: 1 patch 12-16 hours each day. [doses in mg/h: (*Deponit*) [0.2, 0.4]; (*Minitran*) 0.1, 0.2, 0.4, 0.6; (*Nitro Dur*) 0.1, 0.2, 0.3, 0.4, 0.6, 0.8; (*Nitrodisc*) 0.2, 0.3, 0.4; (*Transderm-Nitro*) 0.1, 0.2, 0.4, 0.6, 0.8; (*Nitrocine*) 0.2, 0.4, 0.6].

MANAGEMENT OF CONGESTIVE HEART FAILURE (CHF)

Evaluation/Assessment

- All patients initially presenting with CHF should have an echocardiogram to evaluate left ventricular function. An ejection fraction (EF) of less than 40% indicates *systolic dysfunction*. Heart failure with an EF ≥40% indicates *diastolic dysfunction*.
- Other routine assessment tests: EKG, chest x-ray, CBC, electrolytes, creatinine, albumin, liver function tests, TSH, urinalysis.
- New York Heart Association (NYHA) classification of cardiac disability:

Class I—cardiac disease without resulting limitation of physical activity.
Class II—comfortable at rest, but symptoms (dyspnea/fatigue/palpitations/angina) on regular physical activity.
Class III—comfortable at rest, but symptoms on slight physical activity.
Class IV—symptoms at rest.

CHF Management*

Nonpharmacologic:
• Exercise: Regular walking or cycling for NYHA Class I–III disability.
• Measure weight daily.
• Salt restriction: 3 g sodium diet is reasonable goal; 2 g in severe CHF.
Pharmacologic: for information on drug abbreviations, dosages and side effects not listed below, see **Table 30**, p 61 in the next section.
• Systolic dysfunction. *First line:* Diuretics, ACEI to target levels, eg, (*Captopril*) 50 tid, (*Enalapril*) 20 bid, (*Lisinopril*) 10 bid. Add digoxin (*Lanoxin*) [0.125, 0.25, 0.5; liquid 0.05 mg/mL]; (*Lanoxicaps*) [0.05, 0.1, 0.2], 0.125–0.375 mg qd (monitor serum levels) if CHF is not controlled on diuretics and ACEI. Hydralazine (*Apresoline*) [10, 25, 50, 100] plus isosorbide dinitrate (*Isordil, Sorbitrate*) [5, 10, 20, 30, 40] (initial dose 10 mg tid, target dose 40 mg tid); (*Isordil Tembids*), (*Dilatrate SR*) [40–80 bid] can be used if patient cannot tolerate an ACEI. Recent evidence indicates that carvedilol or angiotensin II receptor blockers improve CHF outcomes (see **Table 30**, p 61).
• Diastolic dysfunction. *First line:* β-Blockers (see **Table 30**, p 61), non-DHP calcium channel blockers. Diuretics should be used judiciously if there is volume overload.
* Source: Adapted from Heart Failure: Evaluation and care of patients with left-ventricular systolic dysfunction. Clinical Practice Guideline # 11 (AHCPR Publication # 1194-0612) 1994.

DYSLIPIDEMIA

Treatment Indications

• Older adults should have dyslipidemia treated if they have overt coronary artery disease (angina, previous MI). Treatment should be considered if they have peripheral or cerebral arterial disease or numerous cardiac risk factors (smoking, hypertension, diabetes, family history, marked obesity, type A personality).
• The treatment threshold for dyslipidemia in older adults without established heart disease should be higher than for those with CAD (see p 57). The appropriate treatment threshold has not been established, but persons with HDL >45 mg/dL, LDL <160 mg/dL, or fewer than 2 cardiac risk factors are at relatively low risk. Some experts use the total cholesterol/HDL ratio of >5 as an indicator of high risk.
Nonpharmacologic Management: A cholesterol-lowering diet should be considered initial therapy for dyslipidemia, and should be used under the following circumstances:
• The patient should be at low risk for malnutrition.
• The diet should be nutritionally adequate, with sufficient total calories, protein, calcium, iron, and vitamins.

- The diet should be easily understood and affordable (a dietitian can be very helpful).

Pharmacologic Management: Target drug treatment according to type of dyslipidemia.

- Elevated LDL, normal triglycerides (TG). HMG-CoA reductase inhibitors, fluvastatin (*Lescol*) 20–40 mg qd/bid [20, 40], lovastatin (*Mevacor*) 10–40 mg qd/bid [10, 20, 40], pravastatin (*Pravachol*) 10–40 mg qd [10, 20], simvastatin (*Zocor*) 5–40 mg qd [5, 10, 20, 40], atorvastatin (*Lipitor*) 10–80 mg qd [10, 20, 40], cervastin (*Baycol*) 0.2–0.3 mg qd in the evening [0.2, 0.3]; monitor CPK and transaminases q3 months for a year; watch for myopathy at higher doses or when used with other antidyslipidemic drug. Alternate: Niacin 100 mg tid to start, increase to 500–1,000 mg tid [25, 50, 100, 250, 500]: monitor for flushing, pruritus, nausea, gastritis, ulcer. Aspirin 325 mg po 30 minutes prior to first niacin dose of the day is quite effective in preventing side effects.
- Elevated TG (>500 mg/dL). Gemfibrozil (*Lopid*) 300–600 mg po bid [300, 600] or niacin.
- Combined (elevated LDL, low HDL, elevated TG). Gemfibrozil or HMG-CoA reductase inhibitor if TG <300 mg/dL. Alternate: Niacin. Conjugated estrogen can also be used in women (see "Osteoporosis," p 36).

HYPERTENSION

Definition/Classification
The Joint National Commission (JNC) VI on Prevention, Detection, Evaluation, and Treatment of High Blood Pressure defines hypertension (HTN) as SBP >140 or DBP >90. In the elderly, many clinicians define HTN as SBP >160 or DBP >90. Isolated systolic HTN (SBP >160 with DBP <90) should be vigorously treated.

Evaluation/Assessment
- After 5 minutes of rest, BP should be measured both standing and sitting.
- Diagnosis is made based on two or more readings at each of two or more visits. Once diagnosis is made, evaluation includes:
  - Collection of cardiac risk factors: Smoking, dyslipidemia, and diabetes are important in older adults.
  - Assessment of end-organ damage: LVH, angina, prior MI, prior coronary revascularization, CHF, stroke or TIA, nephropathy, peripheral arterial disease, retinopathy.
  - Routine laboratory tests: CBC, urinalysis, electrolytes, creatinine, fasting glucose, total cholesterol, HDL cholesterol, and EKG.
  - Think renal artery stenosis if: sudden onset of HTN, sudden rise in BP in previously well-controlled HTN, or HTN despite treatment with three antihypertensives.

Aggravating Factors

Almost all aggravating factors are related to lifestyle: Obesity, excessive alcohol intake, excessive salt intake, lack of aerobic exercise, low potassium intake, low calcium intake, emotional stress, nicotine.

Management

(JNC VI recommendations). BP lowering below 120/80 is not recommended.

Nonpharmacologic Interventions

• Weight reduction: Even a 10-lb weight loss can significantly lower BP.
• Moderation of alcohol intake–limit to 1 oz of ethanol/day.
• Moderation of dietary sodium–watch for volume depletion with diuretic use.
• Aerobic exercise–30–45 minutes most days of the week.
• Adequate dietary potassium intake–fruits and vegetables are the best sources.
• Smoking cessation.
• Adequate calcium and magnesium intake as well as a low-fat diet are recommended for optimizing general health.

Pharmacologic Intervention

• **Table 30,** p 61 lists some commonly used antihypertensives.
• Use antihypertensives carefully in patients with orthostatic BP drop; base treatment decisions on standing BP.
• In the absence of coexisting conditions, a thiazide diuretic or β-blocker can be used as a first-line drug.
• In the presence of coexisting conditions, therapy should be individualized (see **Table 31,** p 66).
• Antihypertensive combinations are listed in **Table 32,** p 67.
• Available dose formulations of oral potassium supplements: [Tablets (mEq)–6.7, 8, 10, 20; liquids (mEq/15 mL)–20, 40; powders (mEq/pack)–15, 20, 25].

Table 30. Oral Antihypertensive Agents

Class/Drug (Trade Name)	Geriatric Dose Range, Total mg/d (Frequency/d)	Formulations	Route of Elimination	Side Effects and Comments
Diuretics				Decrease potassium, sodium, magnesium levels; increase uric acid, calcium, cholesterol (mild), and glucose (mild) levels
Thiazides				
Hydrochlorothiazide (generic, *Esidrix, HydroDIURIL, Oretic*)	12.5–25 (1)	[12.5, 25, liquid 50 mg/mL]	L	(Increased side effects at >25 mg/d)
Chlorthalidone (generic, *Hygroton*)	12.5–25 (1)	[15, 25]	L	(Increased side effects at >25 mg/d)
Indapamide (*Lozol*)	0.625–2.5 (1)	[1.25, 2.5]	L	(Less or no hypercholesterolemia)
Metolazone (*Mykrox*)	0.25–0.5 (1)	[0.5]	L	(Monitor electrolytes carefully)
Metolazone (*Zaroxolyn*)	2.5–5 (1)	[2.5, 5]	L	(Monitor electrolytes carefully)
Loop diuretics				
Bumetanide (generic, *Bumex*)	0.5–4 (1–3)	[0.5, 1, 2]	K	(Short duration of action, no hypercalcemia)
Ethacrynic acid (*Edecrin*)	12.5–50 (1–3)	[25, 50]	K	(Only nonsulfonamide diuretic, ototoxicity)
Furosemide (generic, *Lasix*)	20–160 (1–2)	Capsule [20, 40, 80]; Solution [10, 40/5 mL]	K	(Short duration of action, no hypercalcemia)
Torsemide (*Demadex*)	2.5–50 (1–2)	[5, 10, 20, 100]	LK	
Potassium-sparing				
Amiloride (generic, *Midamor*)	2.5–10 (1)	[5]	LK	Hyperkalemia
Spironolactone (generic, *Aldactone*)	12.5–50 (1–2)	[25, 50]	LK	(Gynecomastia)
Triamterene (generic, *Dyrenium*)	25–100 (1–2)	[50, 100]	LK	

Source: Adapted from JNC VI: The sixth report of the Joint National Committee on Prevention, Detection, Evaluation, and Treatment of High Blood Pressure. *Arch Intern Med.* 1997;157:2413–46. Brackets indicate available dose formulation expressed in milligrams. Listing of side effects is not all-inclusive, and side effects are for the class of drugs except where noted for individual drug (in parentheses). **Bolded** entries indicate agents more suitable for use in geriatric populations.

61

Table 30. Oral Antihypertensive Agents (cont.)

Class/Drug (Trade Name)	Geriatric Dose Range, Total mg/d (Frequency/d)	Formulations	Route of Elimination	Side Effects and Comments
Adrenergic inhibitors				
α-Blockers				
Doxazosin (**Cardura**)	1–16 (1)	[1, 2, 4, 8]	L	Postural hypotension
Prazosin (generic, **Minipress**)	1–30 (2–3)	[1, 2, 5]	L	
Terazosin (**Hytrin**)	1–20 (1)	[1, 2, 5, 10]	LK	
Peripheral agents				
Guanadrel (Hylorel)	5–50 (2)	[10, 25]	K	(Postural hypotension, diarrhea)
Guanethidine (Ismelin)	5–25 (1)	[10, 25]	LK	(Postural hypotension, diarrhea)
Reserpine (generic, Serpasil)	0.05–0.25 (1)	[0.1, 0.25]	LK	(Sedation, depression, nasal congestion, activation of peptic ulcer)
Central α-agonists				
Clonidine (generic, Catapres, Catapres- TTS)	0.1–1.2 (2–3 or patch 1/week)	[0.1, 0.2, 0.3 po or patch]	LK	Sedation, dry mouth, bradycardia, withdrawal hypertension
Guanabenz (Wytensin)	4–16 (2)	[4, 8]	LK	
Guanfacine (Tenex)	0.5–2 (1)	[1, 2]	K	
Methyldopa (generic, Aldomet)	250–2500 (2)	[125, 250, 500; liquid 250 mg/6 mL]	LK	

Source: Adapted from JNC VI: The sixth report of the Joint National Committee on Prevention, Detection, Evaluation, and Treatment of High Blood Pressure. *Arch Intern Med.* 1997;157:2413–46. Brackets indicate available dose formulation expressed in milligrams. Listing of side effects is not all-inclusive, and side effects are for the class of drugs except where noted for individual drug (in parentheses). **Bolded** entries indicate agents more suitable for use in geriatric populations.

Table 30. Oral Antihypertensive Agents (cont.)

Class/Drug (Trade Name)	Geriatric Dose Range, Total mg/d (Frequency/d)	Formulations	Route of Elimination	Side Effects and Comments
β-Blockers				Bronchospasm, bradycardia, heart failure, may mask insulin-induced hypoglycemia
Acebutolol (**Sectral**)	200–800 (1)	[200, 400]	LK	
Atenolol (generic, **Tenormin**)	12.5–100 (1)	[25, 50, 100]	K	
Betaxolol (**Kerlone**)	5–20 (1)	[10, 20]	LK	
Bisoprolol (**Zebeta**)	2.5–10 (1)	[5, 10]	LK	
Carteolol (**Cartrol**)	1.25–10 (1)	[2.5, 5]	K	
Metoprolol (**Lopressor**)	25–200 (2)	[50, 100]	L	
Long-acting metoprolol (**Toprol-XL**)	50–400 (1)	[50, 100, 200]	L	
Nadolol (generic, **Corgard**)	20–160 (1)	[20, 40, 80, 120, 160]	K	
Penbutolol (**Levatol**)	10–20 (1)	[20]	LK	
Pindolol (**Visken**)	5–60 (2)	[5, 10]	K	
Propranolol (generic, **Inderal**)	20–360 (2)	[10, 20, 40, 60, 80, 90; liquid 4/mL, 8/mL]	L	
Long-acting propranolol (**Inderal LA**)	60–320 (1)	[60, 80, 120, 160]	L	
Timolol (generic, **Blocadren**)	10–60 (2)	[5, 10, 20]	LK	
Combined α- and β-Blockers				Postural hypotension, bronchospasm
Carvedilol (**Coreg**)	3.125–25 (2)	[6.25, 12.5, 25]	L	
Labetalol (generic, **Trandate, Normodyne**)	100–600 (2)	[100, 200, 300]	LK	

Source: Adapted from JNC VI: The sixth report of the Joint National Committee on Prevention, Detection, Evaluation, and Treatment of High Blood Pressure. *Arch Intern Med.* 1997;157:2413–46. Brackets indicate available dose formulation expressed in milligrams. Listing of side effects is not all-inclusive, and side effects are for the class of drugs except where noted for individual drug (in parentheses). **Bolded** entries indicate agents more suitable for use in geriatric populations.

63

Table 30. Oral Antihypertensive Agents (cont.)

Class/Drug (*Trade Name*)	Geriatric Dose Range, Total mg/d (Frequency/d)	Formulations	Route of Elimination	Side Effects and Comments
Direct vasodilators				
Hydralazine (generic, *Apresoline*)	40–200 (2–4)	[10, 25, 50, 100]	LK	Headaches, fluid retention, tachycardia (Lupus syndrome)
Minoxidil (generic, *Loniten*)	2.5–50 (1)	[2.5, 10]	K	(Hirsutism)
Calcium antagonists				
Nondihydropyridines				
Diltiazem sustained release (*Cardizem CD, Cardizem SR, Dilacor XR, Tiazac*)	120–360 (1–2)	Once daily [120, 180, 240, 300, 360]; twice daily [60, 90,120]	L	Conduction defects, worsening of systolic dysfunction, gingival hyperplasia (Nausea, headache)
Verapamil sustained release (*Calan SR, Covera-HS, Isoptin SR, Verelan*)	120–480 (1–2)	[120, 180, 240]	L	(Constipation, bradycardia)
Dihydropyridines				
Amlodipine (*Norvasc*)	2.5–10 (1)	[2.5, 5, 10]	L	Ankle edema, flushing, headache, gingival hypertrophy
Felodipine (*Plendil*)	2.5–20 (1)	[2.5, 5, 10]	L	
Isradipine (*DynaCirc*)	5–20 (2)	[2.5, 5]	L	
Isradipine sustained release (*DynaCirc CR*)	5–20 (1)	[5, 10]	L	
Nicardipine (*Cardene*)	60–120 (3)	[20, 30]	L	
Nicardipine sustained release (*Cardene SR*)	60–120 (2)	[30, 45, 60]	L	

Source: Adapted from JNC VI: The sixth report of the Joint National Committee on Prevention, Detection, Evaluation, and Treatment of High Blood Pressure. *Arch Intern Med.* 1997;157:2413–46. Brackets indicate available dose formulation expressed in milligrams. Listing of side effects is not all-inclusive, and side effects are for the class of drugs except where noted for individual drug (in parentheses). **Bolded** entries indicate agents more suitable for use in geriatric populations.

Table 30. Oral Antihypertensive Agents (cont.)

Class/Drug (*Trade Name*)	Geriatric Dose Range, Total mg/d (Frequency/d)	Formulations	Route of Elimination	Side Effects and Comments
Nifedipine sustained release (*Adalat CC, Procardia XL*)	30–120 (1)	[30, 60, 90]	L	
Nisoldipine (*Sular*)	20–60 (1)	[10, 20, 30, 40]	L	
ACE inhibitors				Cough (common), angioedema (rare), hyperkalemia, rash, loss of taste, leukopenia
Benazepril (*Lotensin*)	2.5–40 (1–2)	[5, 10, 20, 40]	LK	
Captopril (generic, *Capoten*)	12.5–150 (2–3)	[12.5, 25, 50]	LK	
Enalapril (*Vasotec*)	2.5–40 (1–2)	[2.5, 5, 10, 20]	LK	
Fosinopril (*Monopril*)	5–40 (1–2)	[10, 20]	LK	
Lisinopril (*Prinivil, Zestril*)	2.5–40 (1)	[2.5, 5, 10, 20, 40]	K	
Moexipril (*Univasc*)	3.75–15 (2)	[7.5, 15]	LK	
Quinapril (*Accupril*)	5–80 (1–2)	[5, 10, 20, 40]	LK	
Ramipril (*Altace*)	1.25–20 (1–2)	[1.25, 2.5, 5, 10]	LK	
Trandolapril (*Mavik*)	1–4 (1)	[1, 2, 4]	LK	
Angiotensin II receptor blockers				Angioedema (very rare), hyperkalemia
Irbesartan (*Avapro*)	75–300 (1)	[75, 150, 300]	L	
Losartan (*Cozaar*)	12.5–100 (1–2)	[25, 50]	LK	
Valsartan (*Diovan*)	40–320 (1)	[80, 160]	L	

Source: Adapted from JNC VI: The sixth report of the Joint National Committee on Prevention, Detection, Evaluation, and Treatment of High Blood Pressure. *Arch Intern Med.* 1997;157:2413–46. Brackets indicate available dose formulation expressed in milligrams. Listing of side effects is not all-inclusive, and side effects are for the class of drugs except where noted for individual drug (in parentheses). **Bolded** entries indicate agents more suitable for use in geriatric populations.

Table 31. Individualizing Antihypertensive Therapy on Basis of Coexisting Conditions

Indication	Thiazide Diuretic	Loop Diuretic	α-Blockers	β-Blockers	Combined α- and β-Blockers	Non-DHP CA	DHP CA	ACEI
Diabetes	+/-[1]	+/-[1]	0	0	+	+	0	++
CHF	+	+	0	-[2]	+	-[2]	-[2]	++[3]
MI	0	0	0	++	0	+	0	++[3]
Angina	0	0	0	+	0	+	+	0
Atrial tachycardia and fibrillation	0	0	0	+	0	+	0	0
Dyslipidemia	-[4]	-[4]	+	-	-	0	0	0
Essential tremor	0	0	0	+	0	0	0	0
Hyperthyroidism	0	0	0	+	0	0	0	0
Osteoporosis	+	0	0	0	0	0	0	0
Prostatism (BPH)	0	0	+	0	0	0	0	0
Renal insufficiency	0	0	0	0	0	0	0	+[5]
Bronchospasm	0	0	0	-	-	0	0	0
Depression	0	0	0	-	-	0	0	0
Urinary urge incontinence	-	-	0	0	0	+	+	0

Source: Adapted from JNCVI: The sixth report of the Joint National Committee on Prevention, Detection, Evaluation, and Treatment of High Blood Pressure. *Arch Intern Med.* 1997;157:2413–2446 and Beard K, Bulpitt C, Mascie-Taylor H, et al. Management of elderly patients with sustained hypertension. *BMJ.* 1992;304(6824):415. Reprinted with permission.

Note: ++ = highly appropriate therapy; + = appropriate therapy; 0 = neither indicated nor contraindicated; - = relative or absolute contraindication; DHP = dihydropyridine; CA = calcium antagonist; ACEI = angiotensin-converting enzyme inhibitor.

1 Low-dose diuretics probably beneficial in DM type 2, high dose relatively contraindicated in DM types 1 and 2.
2 May be beneficial in CHF due to diastolic dysfunction.
3 Appropriate in cases with systolic dysfunction.
4 Low-dose diuretics have a minimal effect on lipids.
5 Use with great caution in renovascular disease.

Table 32. Antihypertensive Combinations

Drug	Trade Name
β-Adrenergic blockers and diuretics	
Atenolol, 50 or 100 mg/chlorthalidone, 25 mg	(*Tenoretic*)
Bisoprolol fumarate, 2.5, 5, or 10 mg/hydrochlorothiazide, 6.25 mg	(*Ziac*)
Metoprolol tartrate, 50 or 100 mg/hydrochlorothiazide, 25 or 50 mg	(*Lopressor HCT*)
Nadolol, 40 or 80 mg/bendroflumethiazide, 5 mg	(*Corzide*)
Propranolol hydrochloride, 40 or 80 mg/hydrochlorothiazide, 25 mg	(*Inderide*)
Propranolol hydrochloride (extended release), 80, 120, or 160 mg/ hydrochlorothiazide, 50 mg	(*Inderide LA*)
Timolol maleate, 10 mg/hydrochlorothiazide, 25 mg	(*Timolide*)
Angiotensin-converting enzyme (ACE) inhibitors and diuretics	
Benazepril hydrochloride 5, 10, or 20 mg/hydrochlorothiazide, 6.25, 12.5, or 25 mg	(*Lotensin HCT*)
Captopril, 25 or 50 mg/hydrochlorothiazide, 15 or 25 mg	(*Capozide*)
Enalapril maleate, 5 or 10 mg/hydrochlorothiazide, 12.5 or 25 mg	(*Vaseretic*)
Lisinopril, 10 or 20 mg/hydrochlorothiazide, 12.5 or 25 mg	(*Prinzide, Zestoretic*)
Angiotensin II receptor antagonists and diuretics	
Losartan potassium, 50 mg/hydrochlorothiazide, 12.5 mg	(*Hyzaar*)
Calcium antagonists and ACE inhibitors	
Amlodipine besylate, 2.5 or 5 mg/benazepril hydrochloride, 10 or 20 mg	(*Lotrel*)
Diltiazem hydrochloride, 180 mg/enalapril maleate, 5 mg	(*Teczem*)
Verapamil hydrochloride (extended release), 180 or 240 mg/ trandolapril, 1, 2, or 4 mg	(*Tarka*)
Felodipine, 5 mg/enalapril maleate, 5 mg	(*Lexxel*)
Other combinations	
Triamterene, 37.5, 50, or 75 mg/hydrochlorothiazide, 25 or 50 mg	(*Dyazide, Maxzide*)
Spironolactone, 25 or 50 mg/hydrochlorothiazide, 25 or 50 mg	(*Aldactazide*)
Amiloride hydrochloride, 5 mg/hydrochlorothiazide, 50 mg	(*Moduretic*)
Guanethidine monosulfate, 10 mg/hydrochlorothiazide, 25 mg	(*Esimil*)
Hydralazine hydrochloride, 25, 50, or 100 mg/hydrochlorothiazide, 25 or 50 mg	(*Apresazide*)
Methyldopa, 250 or 500 mg/hydrochlorothiazide, 15, 25, 30, or 50 mg	(*Aldoril*)
Reserpine, 0.125 mg/hydrochlorothiazide, 25 or 50 mg	(*Hydropres*)
Reserpine, 0.10 mg/hydralazine hydrochloride, 25 mg/ hydrochlorothiazide, 15 mg	(*Ser-Ap-Es*)
Clonidine hydrochloride, 0.1, 0.2, or 0.3 mg/chlorthalidone, 15 mg	(*Combipres*)
Methyldopa, 250 mg/chlorothiazide, 150 or 250 mg	(*Aldoclor*)
Reserpine, 0.125 or 0.25 mg/chlorthalidone, 25 or 50 mg	(*Demi-Regroton*)
Reserpine, 0.125 or 0.25 mg/chlorothiazide, 250 or 500 mg	(*Diupres*)
Prazosin hydrochloride, 1, 2, or 5 mg/polythiazide, 0.5 mg	(*Minizide*)

Approved for initial therapy.
Source: Reprinted from JNCVI: The sixth report of the Joint National Committee on Prevention, Detection, Evaluation, and Treatment of High Blood Pressure. *Arch Intern Med.* 1997;157:2427. Reprinted with permission.

ANTICOAGULATION GUIDELINES

Anticoagulation Indicated in Absence of Active Bleeding or Severe Bleeding Risk

- Atrial fibrillation (valvular or nonvalvular) or pulmonary embolus. Treat indefinitely, target INR 2.0–3.0.
- Deep venous thrombosis (DVT). Treat at least 12 weeks, target INR 2.0–3.0. Treat indefinitely for recurrent DVT.
- Mechanical cardiac valve. Treat indefinitely, target INR 2.5–3.5.
- Prosthetic cardiac valve. Treat 12 weeks, target INR 2.5–3.5.
- Following myocardial infarction. If atrial fibrillation, left ventricular thrombosis or large anterior infarction, target INR 2.0–3.0.
- Initiation of oral anticoagulation with warfarin: Urgent, Day 1 (5–7.5 mg), Day 2 (5–7.5 mg), Day 3 (2–7.5 mg); nonurgent, Day 1 (2–5 mg), Day 2 (2–5 mg), Day 3 (2–5 mg).

Cessation of Anticoagulation Prior to Surgery

- If INR is between 2.0 and 3.0, hold warfarin 4 doses prior to surgery; longer if INR >3.0.
- If patient has a mechanical valve, heparin should be used after warfarin is held prior to surgery.

Table 33. Treatment of Warfarin Overdose

INR	Clinical Situation	Action
>3 and ≤6	No bleeding	Omit next few warfarin doses and restart at lower dose when INR ≤3.0
>6 and ≤10.0	No bleeding	Omit next 2 doses of warfarin; give vitamin K (VK) 2.5 mg po
>6 and ≤10.0	Minor bleeding or no bleeding but in need of rapid reversal for surgery	D/C warfarin; give VK 0.5–1.0 mg IV; repeat VK 0.5 mg IV after 24 hr if INR >3
>10.0 and <20.0	No bleeding	D/C warfarin; give VK 3–5 mg IV; check INR q12h; repeat VK 1–5 mg q12h if INR >6
>10.0 and <20.0	Bleeding	Same as above + fresh frozen plasma (FFP); GET HELP
≥20.0	No bleeding	D/C warfarin; give VK 10 mg IV; check INR q6h; repeat VK q12h as needed; observe very closely for bleeding
≥20.0	Bleeding	D/C warfarin, give VK 10–25 mg IV + FFP; GET HELP

Source: Adapted from Lacy C, Armstrong LL, Ingrim N, Lance LL. *Drug Information Handbook.* 5th ed. Hudson (Cleveland):Lexi-Comp; 1997:1313. Reprinted with permission.

ATRIAL FIBRILLATION (AF)

Evaluation/Assessment

- Causes: *Cardiac disease*–ischemic disease, hypertensive heart disease, valvular disease, cardiomyopathy, CHF, pericarditis, cardiac surgery; *noncardiac disease*–thyrotoxicosis, chronic pulmonary disease, pulmonary emboli, alcoholism, infections.
- Standard testing: EKG, CXR, CBC, electrolytes, creatinine, BUN, TSH, echocardiogram.

Management

- Correct precipitating cause(s).
- Acute-onset AF:
  - D/C cardioversion if compromised cardiac output.
  - If hemodynamically stable with rapid ventricular response (>100 beats/min), lower ventricular rate medically: Options include β-blockers (eg, atenolol [*Tenormin*] 5 mg IV over 5 minutes, may repeat in 10 minutes [0.5 mg/mL], followed by 25–100 mg po qd [25, 50, 100]); calcium channel blockers (eg, verapamil [*Isoptin, Calan*] 5–10 mg IV, may repeat in 15 minutes if no response [2.5 mg/mL], followed by oral sustained release [*Calan SR, Covera-HS, Isoptin SR, Verelan*] 120–480 mg/d; or digoxin [*Lanoxin*] 0.25 mg IV q6h up to 1.0 mg [0.05 mg/mL], followed by 0.125–0.25 mg po qd [0.125, 0.25]).
  - If electric cardioversion or lowering of ventricular rate has not converted patient to sinus rhythm, begin anticoagulation (see "Anticoagulation Guidelines") and seek cardiology consultation for possible pharmacologic or ablative cardioversion.
- Chronic AF:
  - Anticoagulate (see "Anticoagulation Guidelines," p 68) if there are no contraindications.
  - If anticoagulation is contraindicated, begin aspirin 81–325 mg po qd.
  - If electric cardioversion has not been tried in the past, seek cardiology consultation for possible cardioversion.
  - Rate control can be achieved with oral β-blockers, calcium channel blockers, or digoxin (see above for examples and dosages).

DIAGNOSTIC CARDIAC TESTS

Angina/Coronary Artery Disease

- *First line:* ECG, CXR, cardiac enzymes if acute chest pain (troponin, CPK), stress testing.
- Stress testing is a diagnostic cornerstone. The heart is stressed either through exercise (treadmill, stationary bicycle) or, if the patient cannot exercise and/or the ECG is markedly abnormal, with pharmacologic agents (dipyridamole, adenosine, dobutamine). Exercise stress tests can be performed with or without cardiac imaging, while pharmacologic stress tests always include imaging. Imaging can be accomplished by a nuclear isotope (eg, thallium) or echocardiography (ECHO).
- Cardiac catheterization is the gold standard.

Congestive Heart Failure

- *First line:* ECG, CXR, echocardiogram. ECHO provides valuable information about left ventricular size and function, valvular function; difficult to perform in patients with obesity or lung disease.
- Other: Radionuclide ventriculography (RNV). Compared to ECHO, RNV measures ejection fraction more precisely, provides a better evaluation of right ventricular function, and is more expensive.

Palpitations/Presyncope/Syncope

- *First line:* CXR, EKG, 24- or 48-hour rhythm (Holter) monitoring.
- Other: Ambulatory blood pressure monitoring, tilt-table testing.

MUSCULOSKELETAL DISORDERS

SHOULDER PAIN

Differential diagnosis and distinguishing features:

- Rotator cuff tendinitis/subacromial bursitis – Dull ache radiating to upper arm. Painful arc (on abduction 60–120 degrees) is characteristic. Also can be distinguished by applying resistance against active range of motion while immobilizing the neck with hand. Pain on resisted abduction indicates *supraspinatus tendinitis*, pain on resisted external rotation indicates *teres minor* or *infraspinatus tendinitis*; pain when shoulder is passively abducted to 90 degrees without pain on resisted movement indicates *supraspinatus tendinitis* with *subacromial bursitis*.
- Rotator cuff tears – Mild to complete; characterized by diminished shoulder movement. If severe, patients do not have full range of active *or* passive motion. The "drop arm" sign (the inability to maintain the arm in an abducted position) indicates *supraspinatus tear*.
- Bicipital tendinitis – Pain felt on anterior lateral aspect of shoulder; tenderness in the groove between greater and lesser tuberosities of the humerus. Pain is produced on resisted flexion of shoulder, flexion of the elbow, or supination (external rotation) of the hand and wrist with the elbow flexed at the side.
- Frozen shoulder – Loss of passive external (lateral) rotation, abduction, and internal rotation of the shoulder to less than 90 degrees.

BACK PAIN

Differential diagnosis and distinguishing features:

- Unstable lumbar spine – Severe, sudden, short-lasting, frequently recurrent pain often brought on by sudden, unguarded movements. Pain is reproduced upon moving from the flexed to the erect position. Pain is usually relieved by lying supine or on side. Impingement on nerve roots by spurs from facet joints or herniated disks can cause similar complaints although symptoms in these conditions usually worsen as time passes.
- Lumbar spinal stenosis – Symptoms increase on spinal extension (eg, with prolonged standing, walking downhill, lying prone) and decrease with spinal flexion (eg, sitting, bending forward while walking, and lying in the flexed position). Only symptom may be fatigue and/or pain in legs when walking (pseudo-claudication).
- Vertebral compression fracture – Immediate onset of severe pain; worse with sitting or standing; sometimes relieved by lying down.
- Nonrheumatic pain (eg, tumors, aneurysms) – Gradual onset, steadily expanding, often unrelated to position. Night pain when lying down is characteristic. Upper motor neuron signs may be present. Involvement is usually in thoracic and upper lumbar spine.

HIP PAIN

Differential diagnosis and distinguishing features:
- Trochanteric bursitis – Pain in lateral aspect of the hip that usually worsens when patient sits on a hard chair, lies on the affected side, or rises from a chair or bed; pain may improve with walking. On examination, local tenderness over greater trochanter is often present and pain is often reproduced on resisted abduction of the leg or internal rotation of the hip. However, trochanteric bursitis does not produce limited range of motion, pain on range of motion, pain in the groin, or radicular signs.
- Osteoarthritis – "Boring" quality pain in the hip, often in the groin, and sometimes referred to the back or knee with stiffness after rest. On examination, passive motion is restricted in all directions if disease is fairly advanced. In early disease, pain in the groin on internal rotation of the hip is characteristic.
- Hip fracture – Sudden onset usually after a fall, with inability to walk or bear weight, frequently radiating to groin or knee.
- Nonrheumatic pain (eg, referred pain from viscera, radicular pain from the lower spine, avascular necrosis, Paget's disease, metastasis).

Nonpharmacologic Approaches to Osteoarthritis
- Superficial heat: Hot packs, heating pads, paraffin, or hot water bottles (moist heat is better).
- Deep heat: Microwave, shortwave diathermy, or ultrasound.
- Topical analgesics: Linaments, capsaicin cream, ketoprofen gel.
- Biofeedback and transcutaneous electrical nerve stimulation.
- Exercise/physical therapy/occupational therapy: Strengthening, stretching, range of motion, functional activities.
- Weight loss: Especially for low back, hip, and knee arthritis.
- Splinting and assistive devices: Avoid splinting for long periods of time (eg, >6 weeks) since periarticular muscle weakness and wasting may occur.
- Surgical intervention (eg, prosthetic joint replacement).

Pharmacologic Intervention
- Initial drug treatment of choice is acetaminophen [tablet: 80, 325, 500, 650; caplet: 160, 325, 500; elixir: 120/5 mL, 160/5 mL, 167/5 mL, 325/5 mL; liquid: 160/5 mL, 500/15 mL; suppository: 120 mg, 325 mg, 600 mg] not to exceed 4 g/day (ACR). (See **Table 34**, p 72.)
- **Intra-articular injections:** May be particularly effective if monoarticular symptoms (eg, methylprednisolone acetate, triamcinolone acetonide, and triamcinolone hexacetonide) 20–40 mg for large joints (eg, knee, ankle, shoulder), 10–20 mg for wrists and elbows, and 5–15 mg for small joints of hands and feet; often mixed with lidocaine 1% or its equivalent for immediate relief.
- Nonsteroidal anti-inflammatory drugs (NSAIDs, see **Table 34**, p 72), often provide pain relief but have higher rates of side effects. Misoprostol (*Cytotec*) 100–200 mg qid with food [100, 200] may be valuable prophylaxis against NSAID-induced ulcers in high-risk patients.

NOCTURNAL LEG CRAMPS

Stretching exercises may be helpful. Quinine (*Quinamm*) 200–300 mg po hs [200, 260, 300, 325] may reduce the frequency though not the severity of leg cramps. Cinchronism, hemolysis, thrombocytopenia, and visual disturbances are notable side effects.

Table 34. Nonsteroidal Anti-inflammatory Drugs

Drug	Usual Dosage Range for Arthritis	Formulations	Metabolism/ Excretion	Comments
Aspirin*	650 mg every 4–6 hours	[81,325,500,650,975, supp 120,200,300,600]	K	
Extended release (Extended Release Bayer 8 Hour,* ZORprin)	1300 mg tid, 1600 mg to 3200 mg bid			Avoid in renal failure
Aspirin, enteric-coated*	1000 mg qid			
Nonacetylated salicylates (do not inhibit platelet aggregation, less GI and renal side effects, no reaction in ASA-sensitive patients)				
Magnesium salicylate (Magan, Mobidin, Doans)	650–1090 mg tid-qid	[325,545]		
Choline salicylate (Arthropan)	4.8–7.2 g/d divided			
Choline magnesium salicylate – generic or (Trilisate, Tricosal)	3 g/d in 1, 2, or 3 doses	[500,750,1000, liquid 500 mg/mL]	K	
Sodium salicylate*	3.6–5.4 g/d divided doses			
Salicylsalicylic acid (salsalate) – generic or (Disalcid, Mono-Gesic, Salflex)	1500 mg to 4 g/d in 2 or 3 doses	[500,750]	K	Fewer GI side effects
Bromfenac (Duract)	25–50 mg tid-qid	[25 mg]		Recommend use for <10 days
Diclofenac (Voltaren, Cataflam)	50–150 mg/d in 2 or 3 doses	[25,50,75]	L	
Extended release (Voltaren XR)	100 mg/d	[100]	L	
50 mg with misoprostol 200 µg (Arthrotec 50)				
75 mg with misoprostol 200 µg (Arthrotec 75)				
Diflunisal – generic or (Dolobid)	500–1000 mg/d in 2 doses	[250,500]	K	
Etodolac (Lodine)	200–400 mg tid-qid	[200,300,400]	L	Fewer GI side effects
Fenoprofen – or (Nalfon)	200–600 mg tid-qid	[200,300,600]	L	Higher risk of GI side effects
Flurbiprofen (Ansaid)	200–300 mg/d in 2,3 or 4 doses	[50,100]	L	
Ibuprofen – generic or (Motrin, Advil, Nuprin, Rufen)†	1200–3200 mg/d in 3 or 4 doses	[200,400,600,800, susp 100 mg/5 mL]	L	Fewer GI side effects

* Also available without prescription in a lower tablet strength.

Table 34. Nonsteroidal Anti-inflammatory Drugs (cont.)

Drug	Usual Dosage Range for Arthritis	Formulations	Metabolism/Excretion	Comments
Indomethacin – generic or (Indocin)	25–50 mg bid-tid	[25,50, supp 50, susp 25 mg/5 mL]	L	High risk of GI side effects Increased risk of CNS side effects
Extended release – generic or (Indocin SR)	75 mg/d or bid	[75]		Increased risk of CNS side effects
Ketoprofen – generic or (Orudis, Actron)	50–75 mg tid	[12.5,25,50,75]	L	
Sustained release (Oruvail)	200 mg/d	[200]	L	
Ketorolac (Toradol)	10 mg every q4–6h, 15 IM or IV q6h	[10]	K	Duration of use should be limited to 5 days
Meclofenamate sodium – generic or (Meclomen)	200–400 mg/d in 3 or 4 doses	[50,100]	L	High incidence of diarrhea
Nabumetone (Relafen)	1000–2000 mg/d	[500,750]	L	Fewer GI side effects
Naproxen† – generic or (Naprosyn, Aleve)	200–500 mg bid-tid	[200,250,375,500, susp 125 mg/5 mL]	L	
Delayed release (EC-Naprosyn)	375–500 mg bid	[375,500]	L	
Controlled release (Naprelan)	750–1000 mg daily	[375,500]	L	
Naproxen sodium† – generic or (Anaprox)	275 mg or 550 mg bid			
Oxaprozin – generic or (Daypro)	1200 mg/d	[600]	L	
Piroxicam – generic or (Feldene)	20 mg/d	[10,20]	L	Higher rate of GI bleeding
Sulindac – generic or (Clinoril)	150–200 mg bid	[150,200]	L	May have higher rate of renal impairment
Tolmetin – generic or (Tolectin)	600–1800 mg/d in 3 or 4 doses	[200,400,600]	L	

* Also available without prescription in a lower tablet strength.
† Available without a prescription.

73

Table 35. Classification of Tremors

Type	Frequency (Hz)	Associated Condition	Prominent Features	Treatment
Physiologic	8–12	Normal	Low amplitude; ↑ with stress, anxiety, emotional upset, lack of sleep, fatigue, toxins, medications	Treatment of exacerbating factor
Essential	6–12	Familial in 50% of cases	Varying amplitude; common in upper extremities, head, neck; ↑ with antigravity movements, intention, stress, medications	β-Blocker (see p. 63); alternatives are benzodi-azepines (see p. 52), primidone (*Mysoline*) 100 mg qhs start, titrate to 0.5–1.0 g/d in 3–4 divid-ed doses [50, 250; liquid 250 mg/5 mL]
Parkinson's	3–7	Parkinson's disease, parkinsonism	"Pill rolling"; present at rest, ↑ with emotional stress or when examiner calls attention to it; frequently asymmetric	See Parkinson's disease
Cerebellar	3–5	Cerebellar disease	Present only during movement; ↑ with intention; increasing amplitude as target is approached	Symptomatic management

Table 36. Dizziness Classification

Type	Presentation	Common Causes	Tests
Vertigo	Spinning, sensation of abnormal movement	Vestibular disease—benign positional vertigo, labyrinthitis, Meniere's disease, vertebrobasilar insufficiency	Barany maneuver, ear examination, audiometry
Presyncope	Sense of fainting, lightheadedness	Cardiovascular disease—orthostatic hypo-tension, arrhythmia, aortic stenosis	Orthostatic BP measurement, cardiac exam, EKG, Holter monitoring, echocardiography
Disequilibrium	Unsteady gait, imbalance	Vestibular disease or weakness-producing neurologic disorder	Barany maneuver, careful neurologic exam
Nonspecific	Vague sense of lightheadedness	Psychiatric disorders—anxiety (sometimes leading to hyperventilation), depression, substance abuse	Careful psychosocial history; trial of breathing into a paper bag to resolve hyperventilation-induced dizziness

MANAGEMENT OF ACUTE STROKE

Attempt to Diagnose Cause

- Examination: Neurologic (serial examinations), cardiac (murmurs, arrhythmias, enlargement), vascular (carotids and other peripheral pulses), optic fundi.
- Tests: Brain imaging (CT is adequate), EKG, CBC, electrolytes, creatinine, BUN, LFTs, ESR, ABG. Transesophageal echocardiography is preferred over transthoracic echocardiography for detection of cardiogenic emboli. Carotid duplex and transcranial Doppler studies can detect carotid and vertebrobasilar embolic sources, respectively.

Supportive Care

- Control of blood pressure: Do not lower systolic BP if it is <180; higher blood pressures should be lowered *gently;* some experts recommend not lowering systolic BP unless it is over 200.
- Correct metabolic imbalances.
- Monitor and treat for hypoxia.
- Monitor for depression.
- Referral to rehabilitation when medically stable.

Halt or Reverse Progression

- Acute noncardioembolic stroke or TIA: Use aspirin, 325 mg/d (range 81–1300 mg/d) and/or low-dose SQ heparin.
- Cardioembolic stroke: Begin full dose heparin/warfarin anticoagulation starting day 3–7; timing of anticoagulation depends on size of infarct.
- Progressing stroke or crescendo TIAs: Even though there is no evidence that anticoagulation results improve outcomes, some clinicians recommend it in this situation; aspirin would be more conservative therapy. The benefit of emergent thrombolytic therapy is unproven in older adults and should be considered on a case-by-case basis.
- Hemorrhagic stroke: Supportive care.

PARKINSON'S DISEASE

Diagnostic Criteria

- Tremor: Slow frequency, "pill rolling," often occurs at rest, frequently asymmetric.
- Rigidity: Stiffness of limbs or neck, observed with passive range of motion examination; may or may not include cogwheeling.
- Akinesia or bradykinesia: Slowness of movement, difficulty initiating movement.
- Postural changes: Stooped shoulders, slight flexion of back.
- Other features: Micrographia, masked facies, festinating gait, speech abnormalities (hypophonia, dysarthria), disinterest in usual activities.
- Frequently associated conditions: Constipation, orthostatic hypotension, drooling, depression, dementia, anxiety, dry skin, seborrheic dermatitis, urinary retention, urinary incontinence.

Table 37. Drugs for Parkinson's Disease (PD)

Class	Drug (Trade Name)	Initial Dose	Formulations	Route of Elimination	Comments
Dopamine agonists	Carbidopa/levodopa (Sinemet)	1 tablet qd-tid	[10/100, 25/100, 25/250]	L	Mainstay of PD therapy; increase dose as needed; watch for GI side effects, orthostatic hypotension, confusion
	Slow-release carbidopa/levodopa (Sinemet CR)	1 tablet bid	[50/200]	L	Useful at daily dopamine requirement ≥300 mg/d; slower absorption than carbidopa/levodopa; can improve motor fluctuations
Anticholinergics	Benztropine (Cogentin)	0.5 mg qd	[0.5, 1, 2]	L, K	Can provide motoric benefit while minimizing L-dopa therapy; helpful for drooling
	Trihexiphenidyl (Artane)	1 mg qd	[2, 5; elixir 2 mg/5 mL]	L, K	Same as above
MAO B inhibitor	Selegiline (Eldepryl)	5 mg bid (qam and at noon)	[5]	L, K	Symptomatic benefit; not proven to be neuroprotective; expensive
Dopamine reuptake inhibitor	Amantadine (Symmetrel)	100 mg qd-bid	[100, syrup 50 mg/5 mL]	K	Useful in early and late PD; watch closely for CNS side effects, do not discontinue abruptly
Dopamine agonists	Bromocriptine (Parlodel)	1.25 mg bid	[2.5, 5]	L	Titrate over 3–4 weeks to effective dose (15–30 mg/d); very expensive
	Pergolide (Permax)	0.05 mg qd	[0.05, 0.25, 1]	K	Titrate over 3–4 weeks to effective dose (1–4 mg/d); very expensive
	Pramipexole (Mirapex)	0.125 mg tid	[0.125, 0.25, 1.0, 1.5]	K	Titrate over 3–4 weeks to effective dose (1.5–4.5 mg/d)
	Ropinirole (Requip)	0.25 mg tid	[0.25, 0.5, 1, 2, 5]	L	Titrate over 3–4 weeks to effective dose (3–16 mg/d)

Table 38. Commonly Prescribed Antiepileptic Drugs

Agent	Dose (mg)	Target Blood Level (µg/mL)	Formulations	Route of Elimination	Comments
Carbamazepine (Tegretol)	200–600 bid	4–12	[100, 200; susp 100/5 mL]	L, K	Many drug interactions; mood stabilizer; sustained-release preparation (Tegretol XR) also available [100, 200, 400]
Valproic acid (Depakene, Depakote)	250–750 tid	50–100	[125, 250, 500; syrup 250/5 mL]	L	Can cause weight gain; several drug interactions; mood stabilizer
Phenytoin (Dilantin)	250–450 qd	5–20*	[30, 50, 100; susp 30, 125/5 mL]	L	Many drug interactions
Phenobarbital (Luminal)	30–60 bid–tid	20–40	[8, 15, 16, 30, 32, 60; liquid 15/5 mL, 20/5 mL]	L	Many drug interactions; usually not a first-line drug in older adults
Gabapentin (Neurontin)	300–600 tid	Not applicable	[100, 300, 400]	K	Used as adjunct to other agents; adjust dose based on creatinine clearance
Lamotrigine (Lamictal)	100–300 bid	2–4	[25, 100, 150, 200]	L, K	When used with valproic acid, begin at 25 mg qd, titrate to 25–100 mg bid

* Phenytoin is extensively bound to plasma albumin. In cases of hypoalbuminemia or marked renal insufficiency, calculate adjusted phenytoin concentration:

$$C_{adjusted} = \frac{C_{observed}\ (\mu g/mL)}{0.2 \times albumin\ (gm/dL) + 0.1}$$

If creatinine clearance < 10 mL/min, use:

$$C_{adjusted} = \frac{C_{observed}\ (\mu g/mL)}{0.1 \times albumin\ (gm/dL) + 0.1}$$

Obtaining a *free phenytoin level* is an alternate method for monitoring phenytoin in cases of hypoalbuminemia or marked renal insufficiency.

Nonpharmacologic Management
• Patient education is essential and support groups are often helpful. Contact the National Parkinson Foundation, Inc., 1501 NW 9th Ave, Miami, FL 33136 (http://www.parkinson.org/) or the American Parkinson's Disease Association, 710 W 168th St, New York, NY 10032 (http://www.apdaparkinson.com/).
• Exercise program.
• Surgical therapies can be considered for disabling symptoms refractory to medical therapy. Tremor can be improved by thalamotomy or thalamic stimulation. Dyskinesias can be treated by pallidotomy or pallidal and subthalamic stimulation.

SEIZURES

Definition/Classification
• Generalized: All areas of brain affected with alteration in consciousness.
• Partial: Focal brain area affected, not necessarily with alteration in consciousness; can progress to generalized type.

Evaluation/Assessment
• Initial evaluation: *History:* Neurologic disorders, trauma, drug/alcohol use. *Physical examination:* General with careful neurologic. *Routine tests:* CBC, electrolytes, calcium, magnesium, creatinine, BUN, glucose, liver function tests, EKG, head CT, EEG. *As indicated:* Urine toxic/drug screen, oxygen saturation, head MRI, lumbar puncture.
• Common causes: Stroke, advanced dementia, CNS infections, tumor, trauma, metabolic disorders, drug/alcohol withdrawal, toxins, idiopathic.

Management
• Treat underlying causes.
• Antiepileptic drug therapy (see **Table 38**, p 77).
• Virtually all antiepileptics can cause sedation and ataxia.

INFECTIOUS DISEASES

Empiric Treatment of Pneumonia
Presentation can range from subtle (lethargy, anorexia, or confusion) to septic shock or adult respiratory distress syndrome. Pleuritic chest pain, dyspnea, productive cough, chills, or rigors are not consistently present in older patients.

Evaluation/Assessment
• Physical examination: Respiratory rate >20 breaths/minute; low blood pressure; chest sounds may be minimal, absent, or be consistent with CHF. Temperature, 20% will be afebrile.
• CXR: Infiltrate may not be present on initial film if the patient is dehydrated.
• Sputum Gram's stain and culture (optional per ATS guidelines).

- CBC with differential: Up to 50% of patients will have a normal WBC, but 95% will have a left shift.
- BUN, creatinine, electrolytes.
- Blood culture x 2.
- Oxygenation – arterial blood gas or oximetry.

Aggravating Factors
- Age-related changes in pulmonary reserve.
- Comorbid conditions which alter gag reflexes or ciliary transport.
- Alcoholism.
- COPD or other lung disease.
- Heart disease.
- Medications: Immunosuppressants, sedatives, anticholinergic or other agents that dry secretions, agents that decrease gastric pH.
- Altered mental status.
- Nasogastric tubes.
- Malnutrition.

Table 39. Expected Organisms		
Community-Acquired	Nursing Home-Acquired	Hospital-Acquired
Streptococcus pneumoniae	S pneumoniae	Gram-negative bacteria (GNB)
Respiratory viruses	GNB	Anaerobes
Haemophilus influenzae	Staphylococcus aureus	Gram-positive bacteria
GNB	Anaerobes	Fungi
Moraxella catarrhalis	H influenzae	
Legionella spp	Group B streptococcus	
Mycobacterium tuberculosis		
Endemic fungi		

Supportive Management
- Oxygen as indicated.
- Inhaled β-adrenergic agonists.
- Rehydration.
- Chest percussion.
- Mechanical ventilation (if indicated).

Empiric Antibiotic Therapy
- Community-acquired (all via oral route): [Second-generation cephalosporin or trimethoprim/sulfamethoxazole (TMP/SMZ) or β-lactam/β-lactamase inhibitor] ± erythromycin or other macrolide if *Legionella* spp suspected.
- Community-acquired with hospitalization (oral or intravenous route): [Second-, third-, or fourth-generation cephalosporin or β-lactam/β-lactamase inhibitor] ± erythromycin or other macrolide if *Legionella* spp suspected.
- Severe community-acquired with hospitalization (intravenous route initially): Macrolide plus ceftazidime or cefepime or another antipseudomonal agent.
- Nursing home-acquired (intravenous route): [(First- or second-generation

cephalosporin or ureidopenicillin) plus aminoglycoside] ± penicillin G, clindamycin or vancomycin; *or*

Third- or fourth-generation cephalosporin ± aminoglycoside ± penicillin G, clindamycin or vancomycin; *or*

Ureidopenicillin plus aminoglycoside; *or*

Vancomycin plus clindamycin plus aminoglycoside; *or*

For the oral route: See community-acquired pneumonia (all via oral route) ± quinolone.

- Hospital-acquired (intravenous route): [(Third- or fourth-generation cephalosporin) plus clindamycin or penicillin G] ± aminoglycoside; *or* Ureidopenicillin plus aminoglycoside or other antipseudomonal agent; *or* First- or second-generation cephalosporin plus aminoglycoside; *or* Vancomycin plus clindamycin plus aminoglycoside; *or* Ureidopenicillin plus second-generation cephalosporin; *or* β-lactam/β-lactamase inhibitor plus antipseudomonal agent.

For hospital or nursing home-acquired pneumonia, a macrolide, tetracycline, or quinolone may be added or substituted when *Legionella* spp, *Chlamydia pneumoniae*, or *Mycoplasma pneumoniae* is suspected.

Note: The empiric use of vancomycin should be reserved for patients with a serious allergy to β-lactam antibiotics or for patients from environments in which methicillin-resistant *S aureus* is known to be a problem pathogen. For all cases, antimicrobial therapy should be individualized once Gram's stain or culture results are known.

EMPIRIC TREATMENT OF UTI/UROSEPSIS

Definition

Bacteriuria – presence of significant number of bacteria without reference to symptoms

UTI – symptomatic bacteriuria.

Diagnosis is made in the presence of symptoms and one of the following:

- Gram's stain: ≥2 gram-negative organisms/hpf of unspun urine is significant.
- Urine culture: ≥10⁵ cfu/mL.
- Nitrite test: Nitrite positive for a clean-catch specimen.
- Straight catheter collection with growth <10⁵ cfu/mL for men and women.
- For men, any clean-catch urine with growth <10⁵/mL organisms.

Aggravating Factors

- Female gender.
- Abnormalities in function or anatomy of the urinary tract.
- Catheterization or recent instrumentation.
- Limited functional status.
- Comorbid conditions, (eg, diabetes mellitus, benign prostatic hyperplasia).

Assessment and Evaluation (choice is based on presenting symptoms and severity of illness)
• Urinalysis with Gram's stain and culture.
• Blood culture x 2.
• BUN, creatinine, electrolytes.
• CBC with differential.

Expected Organisms
• *Noncatheterized patients:* Most common: *Escherichia coli, Proteus* spp, *Klebsiella* spp, *Providencia* spp, *Citrobacter* spp, and *Enterobacter* spp, and *Pseudomonas aeruginosa* if recent antibiotic exposure, known colonization, or known institutional flora.
• *Nursing-home catheterized: Enterobacter* spp and gram-negative bacteria.

Empiric Antibiotic Management (duration should be at least 7–10 days)
• *Community-acquired or nursing home-acquired cystitis or uncomplicated UTI* (oral route): TMP/SMZ DS, cephalexin, ampicillin, or amoxicillin. Amoxicillin/clavulanic acid should be reserved for patients with sulfur allergy and in settings where β-lactam resistance is known. Fluoroquinolones should be reserved for patients with allergies to sulphur, β-lactams, or in settings where resistance is known.
• *Suspected urosepsis* (intravenous route): Third-generation cephalosporin plus aminoglycoside, aztreonam, or fluoroquinolone ± aminoglycoside. *Vancomycin should be used in patients with severe β-lactam allergy and gram-positive chains or clusters in urine on Gram's stain.*

TREATMENT OF HERPES ZOSTER ("SHINGLES")

Definition
Cutaneous vesicular eruptions followed by radicular pain secondary to the recrudescence of varicella zoster virus.

Clinical Manifestations
• An abrupt onset of pain along a specific dermatome (see "Age-Related Physiologic Changes and Formulas," p 4).
• Macular, erythematous rash after ~3 days which becomes vesicular and pustular (Tzanck cell test positive), crusts over and clears in 10–14 days.
• Complications – postherpetic neuralgia, visual loss or blindness if ophthalmic involvement.

Pharmacologic Management
When started within 72 hours of the appearance of the rash, antiviral therapy decreases the severity and duration of the acute illness and possibly shortens the duration of postherpetic neuralgias.

Antiviral*	Route	Dose	Formulation	Comment†
Acyclovir (*Zovirax*)	Oral	800 mg 5 x a day	[Tablets: 400, 800 mg, Capsules: 200 mg, liquid: 200 mg 15 mL]	Adjust dose when CrCl <50 mL/min.
	IV	10 mg/kg q8h		
	IV for serious illness, ophthalmic infection, or patients who cannot take oral medication.			
Valacyclovir (*Valtrex*)	Oral	1000 mg q8h	[Capsules: 500 mg]	Adjust dose when CrCl <50 mL/min.
	Preferred to po acyclovir; pro-drug of acyclovir with serum concentrations equal to IV.			
Famciclovir (*Famvir*)	Oral	500 mg q8h	[Tablets: 125, 250, 500 mg]	Adjust dose when CrCl <60 mL/min

* Regardless of agent the duration of therapy should be 7 to 10 days.
† The CrCl listed is the threshold below which the dose or frequency should be adjusted. See alternative reference or the drug's package insert for detailed dosing guidelines.

PREVENTION AND TREATMENT OF INFLUENZA (ACIP)

Vaccine Prevention

Yearly vaccination is recommended for all persons ≥65 years and all residents of nursing homes or other residents of residential or long-term care facilities. Nursing home residents admitted during the winter months after the completion of the vaccination program should be vaccinated when they are admitted if they were not already vaccinated.

The influenza vaccine is contraindicated in persons with an anaphylactic hypersensitivity to eggs or any other component of the vaccine. Dose: 0.5 mL IM x 1 in the fall (October/November) for residents in the northern hemisphere.

PHARMACOLOGIC PROPHYLAXIS AND TREATMENT OF INFLUENZA WITH ANTIVIRAL AGENTS

Indications

• Prevention of influenza in persons not vaccinated, who are immunodeficient, or who may spread the virus.
• Prophylaxis for persons vaccinated after an outbreak of influenza A for the 2 weeks required to develop antibodies.
• Reduction in symptoms and duration of illness when started within the first 48 hours of symptoms.

Duration of Antiviral Therapy

Treatment of symptoms: 3–5 days or for 24–48 hours after symptoms resolve. Prophylaxis during an outbreak: Minimum 2 weeks or until ~1 week after the end of the outbreak.

Antiviral	Usual Dose	Dose Adjustment for Renal Function	
Amantadine	100 mg po daily	CrCl (mL/min)	
(*Symmetrel*)		≥30	100 mg daily
		20–29	200 mg 2x/week
		10–19	100 mg 3x/week
		<10	200 mg alternating with 100 mg every 7 days
Rimantadine (*Flumadine*)		100 mg po qd for frail, elderly, and nursing home residents	
		200 mg po qd for adults and others ≥65 years, decrease dose to 100 mg if side effects are experienced.	

Infectious Tuberculosis

Tuberculosis in elderly patients may be the reactivation of old disease or a new infection due to exposure to an infected individual. Treatment recommendations differ and if a new infection is suspected or the patient has risk factors for resistant organisms, bacterial sensitivities must be determined.

Risk Factors for Resistant Organisms
• Exposure to INH-resistant TB or a patient who has failed chemotherapy.
• Previous treatment for TB.
• Homelessness, institutionalization (other than a nursing home), IV drug abuse, and/or HIV infection.
• Origin from geographic regions with a high prevalence of resistance (New York, Mexico, Southeast Asia).
• AFB-positive sputum smears after 2 months of treatment.
• Positive cultures after 4 months of treatment.

Aggravating or Reactivating Factors
• Renal failure.
• Malignancy.
• Diabetes mellitus.
• Malnutrition.
• Corticosteroid use.
• Chronic institutionalization.

Diagnosis
• Purified protein derivative (PPD) with booster: 5-TU subdermal, read in 48–72 hours. Repeat in 1–2 weeks if negative.
• CXR.

Treatment
Indications for Tuberculosis Chemoprophylaxis in Nursing Home Patients
With 5-mm PPD reactivity
• Close contact with active tuberculosis case.
• Known or suspected HIV infection.
• Abnormal CXR with fibrosis consistent with old, cavitated tuberculosis.
With 10-mm PPD reactivity
• Intravenous drug use with no HIV infection.
• Gastrectomy or jejunoileal bypass.

83

- Weight loss ≥10% of ideal body weight.
- Chronic renal failure.
- Diabetes mellitus.
- Immunosuppression.
- Hematologic malignancies (leukemia, lymphoma).

With 15-mm PPD reactivity
- Skin test conversion within 2 years.

Treatment: Isoniazid (INH) 300 mg/day orally or 900 mg orally twice a week (observed) for 6–12 months.

Treatment of active disease when multidrug-resistant tuberculosis is **not** likely: INH 300 mg/day and rifampin 600 mg/day for 9 months.

Treatment of active disease when multidrug-resistant tuberculosis **is** likely: Combination of 4 or 5 of the following: INH 300 mg po or IM qd; rifampin 600 mg po or IV qd or rifabutin; pyrazinamide 15–30 mg/kg/d po tid or qid (max. 2.5 g) or 50–70 mg/kg twice weekly based on LBW; ethambutol (*Myambutol*) 15–25 mg/kg/d po qd; streptomycin 15 mg/kg/d IM q12h. Second-line agents: Capreomycin (*Capastat*) 15 mg/kg IM qd, adjust for CrCl; kanamycin (*Kantrex*) 15 mg/kg/d IM, IV, adjust for CrCl; amikacin (*Amikin*) 15 mg/kg/d IM, IV, adjust for CrCl; cycloserine (*Seromycin*) 250–500 mg po bid; ethionamide (*Trecator-SC*) 250–500 mg po bid; ciprofloxacin (*Cipro*) 500–750 mg po bid, adjust for CrCl; ofloxacin (*Floxin*) 300–400 mg po bid or 600–800 mg po qd; aminosalicylic acid (PAS, *Teebacin*) 4–6 g po bid.

Treatment of Antibiotic Associated Diarrhea

Antibiotic-Associated Pseudomembranous Colitis (AAPMC)

Definition: a specific form of *clostridium difficile* pseudomembranous colitis.

Aggravating factors: almost any oral or parenteral antibiotic and several antineoplastic agents including (cyclophosphamide, doxorubicin, fluorouracil, methotrexate).

Presentation: diarrhea (can be bloody), crampy abdominal pain, leukocytosis, fever (100-105°F), fecal leukocytes, hypovolemia, dehydration, hypoalbuminemia. Symptoms appear a few days after starting to 10 weeks after discontinuing the offending agent.

Diagnosis
- Isolation of *C difficile* or its toxin from symptomatic patient.
- Lower endoscopy, however, lesions may be scattered.

Treatment
- Discontinue the offending agent if possible.
- Metronidazole (*Flagyl*) 250 mg po qid or 500 mg po tid x 10 days or vancomycin 125–500 mg po qid x 10 days.
- Avoid opiates or other agents that will slow gastrointestinal motility.

Recurrence
- Relapse seen in 10% to 20% of patients 1 to 4 weeks after treatment (spore producing organism).
- Retreat with same regimen or use alternative.

Table 40. Antibiotics

Antibiotic Class *Subclass* Individual Antimicrobial	Principal Route of Elimination (%)	Route, Dose, Frequency	Adjust Dose When CrCl Is:*	Formulations
β-Lactams				
Penicillins Amoxicillin (*Amoxil*)	K (80)	PO: 250 mg–1 g q8h	<50 mL/min	[C: 250, 500 mg] [CT: 125, 250 mg] [S: 125, 250 mg/5 mL]
Ampicillin	K (90)	PO: 250–500 mg q6h IM/IV: 1–2 g q4–6h	<30	[C: 250, 500 mg] [S: 125, 250, 500 mg/5 mL; I]
Penicillin G	K L (30)	IV: 3–5 x 106 U q4–6h IM: 0.6–2.4 x 106 U q6–12h	<30	Inj [Procaine for IM]
Penicillin VK	K, L	PO: 125–500 mg q6h		[T: 125, 250, 500 mg] [S: 125, 250 mg/5 mL]
Carbenicillin indanyl sodium (*Geocillin*)	K (80–99)	PO: 382–764 mg q6h	<50	[T: 382 mg]
Ureidopenicillins Mezlocillin (*Mezlin*)	K	IM, IV: 1.5–3 g q4–6h	<30	Inj
Piperacillin (*Pipracil*)	R	IM: 1–2 g q8–12h IV: 2 g q6–8h	<30	Inj
Penicillinase Resistant Nafcillin (*Nafcil*)	L	PO: 250 mg–1g q4–6h IM: 500 mg q4–6h IV: 500 mg–2 g q4–6h	NA	[C: 250 mg] [T: 500 mg] [S: 250 mg/5 mL; I]
Oxacillin (*Bactocill*)	K	PO: 500 mg–1 g q4–6h IM, IV: 250 mg–2 g q4–6h–12h	<10	[C: 250, 500 mg] [S: 250 mg/5 mL; I]

Inj = injectable, T = tablet, C = capsule, CT = chewable tablet, S = liquid.

*The CrCl listed is the threshold below which the dose or frequency should be adjusted. See alternative reference or the drug's package insert for detailed dosing guidelines.

85

Table 40. Antibiotics (cont.)

Antibiotic Class *Subclass* Individual Antimicrobial	Principal Route of Elimination (%)	Route, Dose, Frequency	Adjust Dose When CrCl Is:*	Formulations
Aztreonam (*Azactam*)	K (70)	IM: 500 mg–1 g q8–12h IV: 500 mg–2 g q6–12h	<30	Inj
Meropenem (*Meronem, Merrem IV*)	K (75) L (25)	IV: 1 g q8h	≤50	Inj
Imipenem/Celastatin (*Primaxin*)	K (70)	IM: 500 mg–1 g q8–12h IV: 500 mg–2 g q6–12h	<70	Inj
Amoxicillin–Clavulanate (*Augmentin*)	K	PO: 250 mg q8h, 500 mg q12h, 875 mg q12h	<30	[T: 250, 500, 875 mg] [S: 125, 250 mg/5 mL]
Ampicillin–Sulbactam (*Unasyn*)	K (85)	IM, IV: 1–2 g q6–8h	<30	Inj
Piperacillin–Tazobactam (*Zosyn*)	K	IV: 3.375 g q6h	<40	Inj
Ticarcillin–Clavulanate (*Timentin*)	K, L	IV 3 g q4–6h	<60	Inj
First-Generation Cephalosporins Cefadroxil (*Duricef*)	K (90)	PO: 500 mg–1 g q12h	<50	[C: 500 mg; T: 1 g] [S: 125, 250, 500 mg/5 mL]
Cefazolin (*Ancef, Kefzol*)	K (80–100)	IM, IV: 500 mg–2 g q8h	<55	Inj
Cephalexin (*Keflex*)	K (80–100)	PO: 250 mg–1 g q6h	<40	[C: 250, 500 mg; T: 250, 500 mg, 1 g] [S: 125, 250 mg/5 mL]
Cephalothin (*Keflin*)	K (50–75)	IM, IV: 500 mg–2 g q4–6h	<50	Inj
Cephapirin (*Cefadyl*)	K (60–85)	IM, IV: 1–3 g q6h	<10	Inj

Inj = injectable, T = tablet, C = capsule, CT = chewable tablet, S = liquid.
*The CrCl listed is the threshold below which the dose or frequency should be adjusted. See alternative reference or the drug's package insert for detailed dosing guidelines.

Table 40. Antibiotics (cont.)

Antibiotic Class *Subclass* **Individual Antimicrobial**	Principal Route of Elimination (%)	Route, Dose, Frequency	Adjust Dose When CrCl Is:*	Formulations
Cephradine (*Anspor*)	K (80–90)	PO, IM, IV: 500 mg–2 g q6h	<20	[C: 250, 500 mg] [T: 1 g] [S: 125, 250 mg/5 mL; l]
Second-Generation Cephalosporins				
Cefaclor (*Ceclor*)	K (80)	PO: 250–500 mg q8h	<50	[C: 250, 500 mg] [S: 125, 187, 250, 375 mg/5 mL]
Cefamandole (*Mandol*)	K	IM, IV: 1–3 g q6h	<80	Inj
Cefmetazole (*Zefazone*)	K (85)	IV: 2 g q6–12h	<90	Inj
Cefonicid (*Monocid*)	K	IM, IV: 1 g q24h	<80	Inj
Cefotetan (*Cefotan*)	K (80)	IM, IV:1–3 g q12h or 1–2 g q24h	<30	Inj
Cefoxitin (*Mefoxin*)	K (85)	IM, IV: 1–2 g q6–8h	<50	Inj
Cefpodoxime (*Vantin*)	K (80)	PO: 100–400 mg q12h	<30	[T: 100, 250 mg] [S: 50, 100 mg/5 mL]
Cefprozil (*Cefzil*)	K (60–70)	PO: 250–500 mg q12–24h	<30	[T: 250, 500 mg] [S: 125, 250 mg/5 mL]
Ceftibuten (*Cedax*)	K (65–70)	PO: 400 mg q24h	<50	[C: 400 mg] [S: 180 mg/5 mL]
Cefuroxime axetil (*Ceftin*)	K (66–100)	PO: 125–500 mg q12h IM, IV: 750 mg–1.5 g q6h		[T: 125, 250, 500 mg] Inj
Loracarbef (*Lorabid*)	K	PO: 200–400 mg q12–24h	<50	[C: 200 mg] [S: 100, 200 mg/5 mL]

Inj = injectable, T = tablet, C = capsule, CT = chewable tablet, S = liquid.
*The CrCl listed is the threshold below which the dose or frequency should be adjusted. See alternative reference or the drug's package insert for detailed dosing guidelines.

Table 40. Antibiotics (cont.)

Antibiotic Class *Subclass* Individual Antimicrobial	Principal Route of Elimination (%)	Route, Dose, Frequency	Adjust Dose When CrCl is:*	Formulations
Third-Generation Cephalosporins				
Cefixime (*Suprax*)	K (50%)	PO: 400 mg q24h	<60	[T: 200, 400 mg] [S: 100 mg/5 mL]
Cefoperazone (*Cefobid*)	L, B (Biliary) K (25)	IM, IV: 1–2 g q12h	Adjust in cirrhosis	Inj
Cefotaxime (*Claforan*)	K, L	IM, IV: 1–2 g q6–12h		Inj
Ceftizoxime (*Cefizox*)	K (100)	IM, IV: 500 mg–2 g q4–12h	<80	Inj
Ceftriaxone (*Rocephin*)	K (33–65)	IM, IV: 1–2 g q12–24h	NA	Inj
Fourth-Generation Cephalosporins				
Cefepime (*Maxipime*)	K (85)	IV: 500 mg–2 g q12h	<60	Inj
Aminoglycosides				
Amikacin (*Amikin*)	K (95)	IM, IV: 15–20 mg/kg/d divided q12–24h; 15–20 mg/kg q24–48h		Inj
Gentamicin (*Garamycin*)	K (95)	IM, IV: 2–5 mg/kg/d divided q12–24h; 5–7mg/kg q24–48h		Inj Ophth susp, oint
Netilmicin (*Netromycin*)	K (95)	IM, IV: 2–5 mg/kg/d divided q12–24h; 5–7 mg/kg q24–48h		Inj
Streptomycin	K (90)	IM, IV: 10 mg/kg/d not to exceed 750 mg/d	<50	Inj
Tobramycin (*Nebcin*)	K (95)	IM, IV: 2–5 mg/kg/d divided q12–24h; 5–7mg/kg q24–48h		Inj Ophth susp, oint

Inj = injectable, T = tablet, C = capsule, CT = chewable tablet, S = liquid.
*The CrCl listed is the threshold below which the dose or frequency should be adjusted. See alternative reference or the drug's package insert for detailed dosing guidelines.

88

Table 40. Antibiotics (cont.)

Antibiotic Class *Subclass* Individual Antimicrobial	Principal Route of Elimination (%)	Route, Dose, Frequency	Adjust Dose When CrCl Is:*	Formulations
Macrolides				
Azithromycin (*Zithromax*)	B	PO: 500 mg day 1, then 250 mg qd IV: 500 mg qd	NA	[C: 250 mg] [S: 100, 200 mg/5 mL, 1 g (single-dose packet)] [T: 600 mg]
Clarithromycin (*Biaxin*)	K (20–30)	PO: 250–500 mg q12h	<30	[S: 125, 250 mg/5 mL] [T: 250, 500 mg]
Dirithromycin (*Dynabac*)	L, F (Feces)	PO: 500 mg qd with food	NA	[T: 250 mg]
Erythromycin	L	PO: Base: 333 mg q8h Estolate, stearate or base: 250–500 mg q6–12h Ethylsuccinate: 400–800 mg q6–12h IV: 15–20 mg/kg/d divided q6h	NA	[Base: C, T: 250, 333, 500 mg] [Estolate: 250 mg] [S: 125, 250 mg/5mL] [T: 500 mg] Ethylsuccinate: [S: 100, 200, 400 mg/5 mL] [T: 400 mg] [CT: 200 mg] [Stearate: T: 250 mg, 500 mg] Inj
Quinolones				
Ciprofloxacin (*Cipro*)	K (30–50) B, F (20–40)	PO: 250–750 mg q12h IV: 200–400 mg q12h Ophth: 1–2 drops q2h while awake for 2 days, then 1–2 drops q4h for 5 days	PO: <50 IV: <30	[T: 100, 250, 500, 750 mg] [Ophth solution: 3.5 mg/mL] Inj
Levofloxacin (*Levaquin*)	K	PO, IV: 250–500 mg q24h	<50	[T: 250, 500 mg]
Lomefloxacin (*Maxaquin*)	K	PO: 400 mg q24h	<40	[T: 400 mg]
Norfloxacin (*Noroxin*)	K (30) F (30)	PO: 400 mg q12h Ophth: 1–2 drops q6h	<30	[T: 400 mg] [Ophth 0.3%]

Inj = injectable, T = tablet, C = capsule, CT = chewable tablet, S = liquid.
*The CrCl listed is the threshold below which the dose or frequency should be adjusted. See alternative reference or the drug's package insert for detailed dosing guidelines.

89

Table 40. Antibiotics (cont.)

Antibiotic Class Subclass Individual Antimicrobial	Principal Route of Elimination (%)	Route, Dose, Frequency	Adjust Dose When CrCl Is:*	Formulations
Quinolones (cont)				
Ofloxacin (Floxin)	K	PO, IV: 200–400 mg q12–24h	<50	[T: 200, 300, 400 mg] [Ophth: 0.3%] Inj
Sparfloxacin (Zagam)	L	PO: 400 mg day 1, then 200 mg q24h	<50	[T: 200 mg]
Trovafloxacin (Trovan)	L	PO, IV: 200 mg q24h x 10–14d	NA	[T: 100, 200 mg] [Inj: 200, 300 mg]
Grepafloxacin (Raxar)	L, B	PO: 400–600 mg qd x 10d	NA	[T: 200 mg]
Tetracyclines				
Doxycycline (Vibramycin)	K (25) F (30)	PO, IV: 100–200 mg/d given q12–24h	NA	[C: 100 mg] [S: 50, 100 mg] [S: 25 mg/5 mL] Inj
Minocycline (Minocin)	K	PO, IV: 200 mg stat, 100 mg q12h	NA	[C: 50, 100 mg] [S: 50 mg/5 mL] Inj
Tetracycline	K (60)	PO, IV: 250–500 mg q6–12h	NA	[C: 100, 250, 500 mg] [T: 250, 500 mg] [S: 125 mg/5 mL] [Ophth: Oint, susp] [Topical: Oint, solution]
Other Antibiotics				
Chloramphenicol (Chloromycetin)	L (90)	PO, IV: 50 mg/kg/d given q6h; maximum 4 g/d	NA	[C: 250 mg] [Topical] [Ophth] Inj

Inj = injectable, T = tablet, C = capsule, CT = chewable tablet, S = liquid.
*The CrCl listed is the threshold below which the dose or frequency should be adjusted. See alternative reference or the drug's package insert for detailed dosing guidelines.

Table 40. Antibiotics (cont.)

Antibiotic Class *Subclass* Individual Antimicrobial	Principal Route of Elimination (%)	Route, Dose, Frequency	Adjust Dose When CrCl is:*	Formulations
Clindamycin (*Cleocin*)	L (90)	PO: 150–450 mg q6–8h; maximum: 1.8 g/d IM, IV: 1.2–1.8 g/d given q8–12h; maximum: 3.6 g/d	NA	[C: 75, 150, 300 mg] [S: 75 mg/5 mL] [Cream, vaginal: 2%] [Gel, topical: 1%]
Co-trimoxazole (TMP/SMZ, *Bactrim*)	K, L	Doses based on the trimethoprim component: PO: 1 DS tablet q12h IV: Sepsis: 20 TMP/kg/d given q6h	≤50	[T: SMZ 400 mg, TMP 80 mg] [DS: SMZ 800 mg, TMP 160 mg] [S: SMZ 200 mg, TMP 40 mg/5 mL] Inj
Nitrofurantoin (*Macrodantin*)	L (60) K (40)	PO: 50–100 mg q6h	Do not use if CrCl <40	[C: 25, 50, 100 mg] [S: 25 mg/5 mL]
Vancomycin (*Vancocin Hydrochloride*)	K (80–90)	PO: *C. difficile:* 125–500 mg q6–8h; IV: 500 mg–1 g q8–24h		[C: 125, 250 mg] Inj
Antifungals				
Amphotericin B (*Fungizone*)	K	IV: Test dose: 1 mg infused over 20–30 minutes. If tolerated, the initial therapeutic dose is 0.25 mg/kg. The daily dose can be increased by 0.25-mg/kg increments on each subsequent day until the desired daily dose is reached. Maintenance dose: IV: 0.25–1 mg/kg/d or 1.5 mg/kg qod; do not exceed 1.5 mg/kg/d.	Adjust dose if decreased renal function due to the drug or give every other day.	[C, L, topical: 3%] Inj [Susp, as lipid complex: 100 mg/20 mL]

Inj = injectable, T = tablet, C = capsule, CT = chewable tablet, S = liquid.
*The CrCl listed is the threshold below which the dose or frequency should be adjusted. See alternative reference or the drug's package insert for detailed dosing guidelines.

91

Table 40. Antibiotics (cont.)

Antibiotic Class / *Subclass* / Individual Antimicrobial	Principal Route of Elimination (%)	Route, Dose, Frequency	Adjust Dose When CrCl Is:*	Formulations
Antifungals (cont)				
Fluconazole (*Diflucan*)	K (80)	PO, IV: First dose 200–400 mg, then 100–400 mg qd for 14 days to 12 weeks depending on indication. Vaginal candidiasis: 150 mg as a single dose.	<50	[T: 50, 100, 150, 200 mg] [S: 10 and 40 mg/mL] Inj
Flucytosine (*Ancobon*)	K (75–90)	PO: 50–150 mg/kg/d divided q6h	<50	[C: 250, 500 mg]
Griseofulvin (*Fulvicin P/G, Grifulvin V*)	L	PO: Microsize 500–1000 mg/d in single or divided doses. Ultramicrosize: 330–375 mg/d in single or divided doses. Duration based on indication.	NA	Microsize: [C: 125, 250 mg] [S: 125 mg/5 mL] [T: 250, 500 mg] Ultramicrosize: [T: 125, 165, 250, 330 mg]
Itraconazole (*Sporanox*)	L	PO: 200–400 mg daily, doses >200 mg/d should be divided. Life-threatening infections: Loading dose: 200 mg tid (600 mg/d) should be given for the first 3 days of therapy.	NA	[C: 100 mg] [S: 100 mg/10 mL]
Ketoconazole (*Nizoral*)	L, F	PO: 200–400 mg qd. Shampoo: Twice weekly for 4 weeks with at least 3 days between each shampoo. Topical: Apply qd-bid.	NA	[C: 2%] [Shampoo: 2%] [T: 200 mg]
Miconazole (*Monistat IV*)	L, F	IT: 20 mg every 1–2 days. IV: Initial: 200 mg, then 1.2–3.6 g/d divided q8h for up to 20 weeks.	NA	Inj

Inj = injectable, T = tablet, C = capsule, CT = chewable tablet, S = liquid.
*The CrCl listed is the threshold below which the dose or frequency should be adjusted. See alternative reference or the drug's package insert for detailed dosing guidelines.

RESPIRATORY DISEASES

ALLERGIC RHINITIS

Definition
The most common atopic disorder; symptoms include rhinorrhea, sneezing, and irritated eyes, nose and mucous membranes; symptoms may be seasonal, but in older people are more often perennial. Postnasal drip, mainly from chronic rhinitis, is the most common cause of chronic cough.

Therapy
- Nonpharmacologic: Avoid allergens, eliminate pets and their dander; dehumidification to reduce molds; reduce outdoor exposures during pollen season; reduce house dust mites by encasing pillows and mattresses; arachnocides reduce mites; household electrostatic particle precipitators are controversial.
- Pharmacologic: (see **Table 41**, p 95).
  - Antihistamines reduce sneezing and rhinorrhea, not congestion; better in seasonal and allergic than perennial rhinitis; best to start before allergy season.
  - Decongestants reduce nasal congestion; topical therapy is more rapid and more effective than systemic; topical use for more than a few days produces rhinitis medicamentosa (ie, rebound rhinitis). Main uses: to permit topical steroid administration; to facilitate sleep during severe attacks.
  - Cromolyn sodium works best when given before seasonal symptoms begin or before episodic exposure.
  - Glucocorticoids are the most potent therapy for allergic rhinitis; topical preparations do not produce significant systemic effects; also effective in perennial and vasomotor rhinitis.
  - Ipratropium reduces rhinitis, not congestion.

CHRONIC OBSTRUCTIVE PULMONARY DISEASE

Definition
A spectrum of chronic respiratory diseases characterized by cough, sputum production, dyspnea, airflow limitation, impaired gas exchange, and frequent pulmonary infection.

Therapy
Stepped approach, add additional steps when symptoms inadequately controlled, discontinue agents if no improvement with a given agent (see **Table 42**, p 97 and **Table 43**, p 98). Smoking cessation is essential at any age. Indications for long-term oxygen therapy are given in **Table 44**, p 100.

ASTHMA

Definition
Chronic inflammatory disorder of the airways; may be triggered by viruses, allergens, tobacco smoke, air pollution, exercise, emotional distress, chemicals.

Characteristics
Wheezing, cough, shortness of breath, chest tightness, and reversible and variable peak expiratory flow (PEF). Asthma can present at any age; in old age, cough is a common presentation.

Therapy
- Nonpharmacologic: Avoid triggers; educate patients on disease management, use of metered dose inhalers (MDIs) and peak flow meters.
- Pharmacologic: In a stepped approach based on severity of presenting symptoms; when symptoms are controlled for 3 months, attempt a gradual stepwise reduction; if control is not achieved, step up, but first review medication technique, compliance, and avoidance of triggers (see **Tables 43, 44,** and **45,** p 98, 100, and 101).

PULMONARY EMBOLISM (PE)

Symptoms
Classic triad—dyspnea, chest pain, hemoptysis— occurs in ≤20% of cases. Consider PE in patients with any of the following: chest pain, shortness of breath, tachycardia, hypoxia, hypotension, hemoptysis, or syncope; dyspnea may resolve spontaneously after PE.

Diagnosis
Ventilation-perfusion (V-P) lung scans: normal scan reduces probability of PE to 4% in a high-risk setting and effectively excludes PE in an average or low probability setting; a high probability scan has a sensitivity of 41% and positive predictive value of 87% in high-risk settings. With low risk of complications and a high probability scan, begin treatment for PE; intermediate or low probability scans are nondiagnostic and are not sufficient to exclude PE.
- Plasma d-dimer <500 μg/L effectively excludes PE in the setting of nondiagnostic V-P_R scan.
- Ultrasound of the lower limbs when positive for DVT warrants anticoagulation without resorting to angiography.
- Spiral-chest CT or MRI angiography shows promise as noninvasive diagnostics in circumstances that would otherwise warrant angiography.
- Pulmonary angiography is most accurate, false negative is 0–10%; complication rate 5%; mortality 1–4/1000.

Therapy
- Pharmacologic: Standard therapy for PE remains IV heparin followed by warfarin. There is evidence for the utility and safety of subcutaneous low-molecular-weight heparins for the treatment of both DVT and PE. Thrombolytic therapy is indicated and effective in massive PE.
  - Heparin: (see **Table 46,** p 102). Mix infusion 100 units/mL in D5W; metabolism liver and kidney; half life of anticoagulation effect 1.5 hours.

Table 41. Drug Therapy for Allergic/Perennial Rhinitis

Drug Type	Geriatric Dose (for each nares)	Formulations	Half-Life Geriatric	Side Effects
H₁-Receptor Antagonists/Antihistamines				
First Generation				
Chlorpheniramine (*Chlor-Trimeton*)	8–12 mg bid	Tablets 4, 8, 12 mg	20 hrs, longer with renal dysfunction	Sedation, dry mouth, constipation, confusion, urinary retention. (May be caused by all agents in this class.)
Hydroxyzine (*Atarax*)	25–30 mg bid	Tablets 10, 25, 50 mg	30 hrs	
Diphenhydramine (*Benadryl*)	25–50 mg bid	Tablets 25, 50 mg Elixir 12.5 mg/mL	13.5 hrs	
Second Generation – Low or nonsedating				
Astemizole (*Hismanal*)	10 mg/day	Tablets 10 mg	24 hrs	Astemizole can cause QT-prolongation and is contraindicated with macrolide antibiotics, ketoconazole, itraconazole or nefazodone. Same may apply to others in this class.
Loratadine (*Claritin*)	SR not recommended 5 mg qd-bid	Tablets 10 mg	Metabolites >12 days Wide variation	
Cetirizine (*Zyrtec*)	5 mg/day (max)	Tablets 5, 10 mg	Prolonged	
Levocabastine (*Livostin*)	Topical: 2 puffs each nares bid-qid	Microsuspension 0.5 mg/mL	40 hrs	
Fexofenadine (*Allegra*)	60 mg bid	Tablets 60 mg	14 hrs	
Decongestants				
Phenylpropanolamine	25 mg po q 4 hr SR 75 mg po bid	Tablets 25, 50 mg	6 hrs	Caution with high BP, diabetes, hyperthyroidism, glaucoma. Chronic use may cause high BP.
Pseudoephedrine (*Sudafed*, and combinations)	60 mg po q 4-6 hr SR 120 mg po bid	Tablets 30, 60, SR 120 mg Elixir 30 mg/5 mL	2–16 hrs—Varies with urine pH	Arrhythmia, insomnia, anxiety, restlessness.

Table 41. Drug Therapy for Allergic/Perennial Rhinitis (cont.)

Drug Type	Geriatric Dose (for each nares)	Formulations	Half-Life Geriatric	Side Effects
Nasal Steroids				
Beclomethasone (Vancenase, Beconase)	1 spray bid/tid/qid	Topical spray 16 g [80 sprays]	Rapid absorption, hepatic metabolism	Nasal burning, sneezing, irritation, bleeding; septal perforation (rare); fungal overgrowth is rare. Applies to all nasal steroids
Budesonide (Rhinocort)	2 sprays bid or 4 qd	7g [200 sprays]		Applies to all nasal steroids
Dexamethasone (Decadron)	2 sprays bid/tid	25 mL		
Flunisolide (Nasalide)	2–4 sprays bid/tid	25 mL [200 sprays]		
Fluticasone (Flonase)	2 sprays q day	16 g [120 sprays]		
Triamcinolone (Nasacort)	2–4 sprays q day	10 g [100 sprays]		
Other				
Ipratropium	2 sprays bid-qid	.03, .06% solution	1.6 hr	Epistaxis, nasal irritation, URI, sore throat, nausea. Caution: Do not spray in eyes.

- Warfarin (*Coumadin, Panwarfin, Saturin, Carfin, Wartilone*) [1,2,2.5,3,4, 5,6,7.5,10 mg] begin anticipated maintenance dose at the same time as heparin. Loading dose is not necessary and increases risk of hemorrhage (see "Cardiovascular Disease," p 56).
- Low-molecular-weight heparins–enoxaparin (*Lovenox*) 1 mg/kg sc bid; renal excretion, half-life 4.5 hours; or dalteparin (*Fragmin*) 120 AntiXa units/kg sc bid; renal excretion, half-life 3–4 hrs. Effects may be prolonged in renal failure. No geriatric dose adjustment is necessary. Other low-molecular-weight heparins may be effective but have not received FDA approval.

• Acute massive PE, defined as filling defects in 2 or more lobar arteries, or the equivalent, by angiogram, associated with hypotension, or severe hypoxia, or high pulmonary pressures on echocardiogram should usually be treated with thrombolytic therapy within 48 hours of onset. Risk of hemorrhage probably increases with age and with greater body mass index.
- Streptokinase (*Streptase, Kabikinase*) 250,000 U over 30 min and 100,000 U IV/h for 24 hours; liver metabolism, biological half-life 1.3 hours; adverse reactions hemorrhage, hypotension, hallucination, agitation, confusion, rash, serum sickness.
- Urokinase (*Abokinase*) 4400 IU/kg in 15 mL of D5W or NS over 30 min, then 4400 IU/kg in 15 mL solution per hour for 12 hours, not to exceed 200 mL total volume; half life 20 min; liver metabolism; side effects include hemorrhage, fever, platelet aggregation.

Table 42. Modified from ATS Guidelines–Step-by-Step COPD Therapy		
Step	**Symptom/Severity**	**Therapy**
1	Mild intermittent	β_2-agonist MDI 1–2 puffs q2–6 hrs prn not to exceed 8–12 puffs/24 hrs.
2	Mild to moderate continuing symptoms	Ipratropium MDI 2–6 puffs q 6–8 hrs; plus β_2-agonist 1–4 puffs qid prn or routine.
3	If response to step 2 suboptimal or if symptoms progress	Theophylline-SR 200 mg bid or 400 mg at hs for nocturnal bronchospasm; and/or albuterol 4–8 mg bid or hs; and or mucokinetic agent.
4	If symptoms persist	Oral steroids (eg, prednisone up to 40 mg/d) for 10–14 days; no improvement stop the steroid; if improvement taper to lowest effective dose, alternate day dosing or steroid MDI.
5	For severe exacerbation	↑ (β_2-agonist), eg, MDI 6–8 puffs q 1/2–2 h or inhalant solution, unit dose every 1/2–2 h, or sc epinephrine or terbutaline, 0.1–0.5 mL, **and/or** ↑ ipratropium MDI 6–8 puffs q 3–4 h or inhalant solution 0.5 mg q 4–8 hrs, **and** theophylline IV calculated to bring serum level to 10–12 µg/mL, **and** methylprednisolone IV 50–100 mg STAT and q 6–8 hrs; taper as soon as possible **and add:** an antibiotic, if indicated; a mucokinetic agent if sputum is very viscous.

Source: From *Am J Respir Crit Care Med*. 1995;152:S77–S121. Official Journal of the American Thoracic Society © American Lung Association. Reprinted with permission.

Table 43. Asthma and COPD Medications

Agents	Dose	Half-life	Metabolism	Side Effects
Anticholinergics				
Ipratropium (Atrovent)	MDI with spacer 2–6 puffs qid	2–4 hr	Lung; poorly absorbed	Dry mouth, bitter taste
Short-acting β₂ – agonists				
Albuterol (Ventolin, Proventil)	2–6 puffs q 4–6 hours	2–7 hr	Liver	Tremor, nervousness, headache, palpitation, tachycardia, cough, hypokalemia. Caution: use half doses in persons with known or suspected coronary disease. (This applies to other agents in this class.)
Bitolterol (Tornalate)	1–3 puffs q 4–6 hours		Liver	
Isoetharine (Bronkosol, Bronkometer)	.25–.5 mL of 1% soln. 2 mL NS by neb q1–4 hr; inhaler 1–2 puffs q4hr		Liver	
Metaproterenol (Alupent, Metaprel)	.3mL 5% soln. q 4 hr; inhaler 2–3 puffs q 3–4 hr, oral forms also		Liver	
Pirbuterol (Maxair)	2–3 puffs q 4–6 hours	2–3 hr	Liver	
Long-acting β₂ –agonists				
Salmeterol (Serevent)	2 puffs bid	3–4 hr	Liver	Tremor, nervousness, headache, palpitation, tachycardia, cough, hypokalemia. Caution: use half doses in persons with known or suspected coronary disease. Not for acute exacerbation.
Brethaire-inhaler in US	2 puffs q 4 – 6 hours	20 hr	Liver	
Terbutaline (Brethine-sc) (Brethine, Brycanyl-tabs)	.25 mg 2.5–5 mg tid [2.5, 5]	20 hr	Liver	Tremor, nervousness, headache, palpitation, tachycardia, cough, hypokalemia. Caution: use half doses in persons with known or suspected coronary disease. Not for acute exacerbation.

Table 43. Asthma and COPD Medications (cont.)

Agents	Dose	Half-life	Metabolism	Side Effects
Long-acting theophyllines				
(*Quibron-T/Sr*)	300–400 mg/d 300 mg bisect, trisect [tabs]	6–13 hr	Liver; clearance reduced by 30% in older patients. Caution: start max 400 mg/day and follow blood levels	Atrial arrhythmias, seizures, increased gastric acid secretion, ulcer, reflux, diuresis. Applies to all long-acting theophyllines.
(*Uniphyl, Theo-24*)	400 mg po q day [tabs 100, 200, 300, 400 mg]	6–13 hr	Liver; clearance reduced by 30% in older patients. Caution: start max 400 mg/day and follow blood levels	
(*Theo-dur, Slo-bid*)	100–200 mg po bid [tabs 100, 200, 300, 450 mg]	6–13 hr	Liver; clearance reduced by 30% in older patients. Caution: start max 400 mg/day and follow blood levels	
Corticosteroids				
Oral Prednisone (*Deltasone, Orasone*)	20 mg po bid [tabs: 1, 2.5, 5, 10, 20, 50; elixir 5 mg/5 mL]	3 hr	Liver	Leukocytosis, thrombocytosis, sodium retention, euphoria, depression, hallucination, cognitive dysfunction; other effects with long-term use.
Inhaled Beclomethasone (*Vanceril, Beclovent*)	2–4 puffs qid [42, 84 μg/puff, max 840 mg 1 d]	3 hr	Liver; trivial systemic absorption	Nausea, vomiting, diarrhea, abdominal pain; oropharyngeal thrush. Applies to all inhaled steroids.
Budesonide (*Pulmicort*)	1–2 puffs qid [100, 200, 400 μg/puff; 400–1600 μg/d]	2–3 hr	Liver	
Flunisolide (*Aerobid*)	2–4 puffs bid [250 μg/puff]	3–5 hr	Liver	
Fluticasone (*Flovent*)	1 puff [44, 110, 220 μg/puff]	3 hr	Liver	
Triamcinolone (*Azmacort*)	2 puffs tid-qid or 4 puffs bid [100 μg]	2–5 hr	Liver	
Dexamethasone (*Dexacort*)	3 puffs tid-qid [100 μg/puff]	3–6 hr	Liver	

Table 43. Asthma and COPD Medications (cont.)

Agents	Dose	Half-life	Metabolism	Side Effects
Other Asthma Medications				
Cromolyn sodium (*Intal*)	2–4 puffs or 20 mg caps inhaled qid	1–2 hr	Liver/kidney	Use MDI with caution in coronary disease or arrhythmia due to propellent in the product
Nedocromil (*Tilade*)	2 puffs qid	2 hr	Excreted unchanged urine and feces	Bitter taste, headache, dizziness, sore throat, cough, chest tightness
Zafirlukast (*Accolate*)	20 mg po bid 1 hr before or 2 hrs after meals	10 hr	Liver; reduced by 50% >65 yrs	Headache, somnolence, dizziness, nausea, diarrhea, abdominal pain, increased LFTs, fever
Zileuton (*Zyflo*)	600 mg po qid	2.5 hr	Liver	Dizziness, insomnia, nausea, abdominal pain, abnormal LFTs, myalgia

Table 44. Indications for Long-Term Oxygen Therapy

Absolute
PaO_2 ≤55 mm Hg or SaO_2 ≤88%

In presence of cor pulmonale
- PaO_2 55–59 mm Hg or SaO_2 ≥89%
- ECG evidence of "P" pulmonale, hematocrit >55%, congestive heart failure

Only in specific situations
- PaO_2 ≥60 mm Hg or SaO_2 ≥90%
- With lung disease and other clinical needs, such as sleep apnea with nocturnal desaturation not corrected by CPAP

If the patient meets criteria at rest, O_2 should also be prescribed during sleep and exercise, appropriately titrated.

If the patient is normoxemic at rest but desaturates during exercise or sleep (PaO_2 ≤55 mm Hg), O_2 should be prescribed for these indications.

Also consider nasal CPAP or BiPAP

CPAP = continuous positive airway pressure; BiPAP = bilevel positive airway pressure.
Source: *Am J Respir Crit Care Med.* 1995;152:S92. Official Journal of the American Thoracic Society © American Lung Association. Reprinted with permission.

Table 45. Asthma Therapy

Step	Symptoms/Severity Day/Night	PEF	Quick-Relief Therapy	Long-Term Prevention
1 Intermittent Asthma	Symptoms <1/week; night symptoms: ≤2 times/month	Normal PEF between attacks. PEF ≥80% predicted. Variability <20%.	Short-acting: Inhaled β₂-agonist <1/week. Treatment will depend on severity of attack. Inhaled β₂-agonist or cromolyn before exercise or allergen exposure.	None needed.
2 Mild Persistent Asthma	Symptoms >1/week, but <1/day; Night symptoms: >2 times/month	PEF ≥80% predicted. Variability 20-30%.	Short-acting: Inhaled β₂-agonist as needed but not to exceed 3-4 times/day.	Daily meds: Either inhaled corticosteroid, 200-500 µg, cromolyn, nedocromil, or theophylline-SR. If needed, increase inhaled corticosteroids up to 800 µg or add either long-acting inhaled β₂-agonist, theophylline-SR, or oral β₂-agonist.
3 Moderate Persistent Asthma	Daily symptoms: Requiring short-acting β₂-agonist prn daily. Attacks affect activity. Night symptoms: >1 time/week	PEF >60%–<80% predicted. Variability >30%.	Short-acting: Inhaled β₂-agonist prn for symptoms, not to exceed 3-4 times/day.	Daily meds: Inhaled corticosteroids, ≥800-2,000 µg and long-acting bronchodilator: either inhaled β₂-agonist, theophylline-SR, or oral β₂-agonist.
4 Severe Persistent Asthma	Continuous symptoms: Limited physical activity. Frequent night symptoms.	≤60% predicted. Variability >30%.	Short-acting: Inhaled β₂-agonist as needed for symptoms.	Daily meds: Inhaled corticosteroid, 800-2,000 µg or more, and either long-acting inhaled β₂-agonist, or theophylline-SR, and/or oral β₂-agonist, and oral corticosteroid.

PEF = peak expiratory flow.
Source: Adapted from: *NHLBI/WHO Guide for Asthma Management and Prevention, 1995.* Reprinted with permission.

Table 46. Weight-Based Heparin Dosage	
Initial	80 U/kg bolus = _____ U (not to exceed 10,000 U) 18 U/kg/h = _____ U/h (not to exceed 1500 U)
PTT < 35	80 U/kg bolus = _____ U Increase drip 4 U/kg/h = _____ U/h
PTT 35 to 45	40 U/kg bolus = _____ U Increase drip 2 U/kg/h = _____ U/h
PTT 46 to 70	No change
PTT 71 to 90	Reduce drip 2 U/kg/h = _____ U/h Hold heparin for 1 h Reduce drip 3 U/kg/h = _____ U/h

NOTE: Order a partial thromboplastin time (PTT) 6 hours after any dosage change, adjusting heparin infusion by the sliding scale until PTT is therapeutic (46 to 70 seconds). When two consecutive PTTs are therapeutic, order PTT (and readjust heparin drip as needed) every 24 hours. U = units.
SOURCE: Adapted from Raschke RA, Reilly BM, Guidry JR, et al. Weight-based heparin dosing nomogram compared with a standard care nomogram. *Ann Intern Med.* 1993;119(9):874. Reprinted with permission.

GASTROINTESTINAL DISEASES

GASTROESOPHAGEAL REFLUX DISEASE (GERD)

Definition
The retrograde movement of the gastric contents in the esophagus.

Contributing Factors
Incompetent lower esophageal sphincter, transient relaxations of the sphincter, and compromise of other antireflux mechanisms.

Evaluation and Assessment
• Endoscopy – if symptoms persist despite initial management, atypical presentation.
• Radiologic evaluation.
• 24-hour pH monitoring.
• Esophageal manometry.

Aggravating Factors
Chocolate, alcohol, fat, tobacco, caffeine (?)

Management
Nonpharmacologic
• Elevate head of the bed (6–8 inches).
• Avoid tight-fitting clothes.
• Weight loss.
• Avoid alcohol.
• Stop smoking.
• Avoid eating immediately before bedtime.
• Dietary changes – avoid pepper and spearmint, chocolate, spicy or acidic foods.

Table 47. Pharmacologic Management of GERD

Drug	Initial Oral Dose	Maximum Dose	Formulations	Excretion/Metabolism
H₂ Antagonists				
Cimetidine (*Tagamet*)	200,* 400, or 800 mg BID	1.5–2.0 times initial dose	[Infusion NS 300 mg/50 mL; injection 150 mg/mL; liquid 300 mg/5mL with alcohol 2.8%; tablets 200,* 300, 400, 800 mg]	K, L
Ranitidine (*Zantac*)	75* or 150 mg bid	1.5–2.0 times initial dose	[Capsule (*GELdose*) 150 mg, 300 mg granules, effervescent (*EFFERdose*) 150 mg; infusion in NaCl 0.45% 1 mg/mL; injection 25 mg/mL; syrup 15 mg/mL; tablet 75,* 150, 300 mg; tablet, effervescent (*EFFERdose*) 150 mg]	K, F
Famotidine (*Pepcid*)	10* or 20 mg bid	1.5–2.0 times initial dose	[Infusion in NS: 20 mg/50 mL; injection 10 mg/mL; oral suspension 40 mg/5mL; film-coated tablet 10,* 20, 40 mg]	K
Nizatidine (*Axid*)	75* or 150 mg bid	1.5–2.0 times initial dose	[Capsule 150; tablet 75 mg]	K
Mucosal Protective Agents				
Sucralfate (*Carafate*)	1 g qid, pc and hs	4 g/day	[Oral suspension 1g/10; tablet 1g]	F, K
Prokinetic Agents				
Metoclopramide (*Reglan*)	5 mg qid, ac and hs	15 mg/day	[Injection 5 mg/mL; syrup, sugar free: 5 mg/5 mL; tablet 5 mg, 10 mg]	K, F
Cisapride (*Propulsid*)	10 mg qid	20 mg qid	[Tablet scored 10, 20 mg; suspension, oral 1 mg/mL]	L
Bethanechol (*Urecholine*)	25 mg qid	50 mg qid	[Injection 5 mg/mL; tablet 5, 10, 25, 50 mg]	Unknown
Proton-Pump Inhibitors				
Lansoprazole (*Prevacid*)	30 mg qd x 8 weeks	60 mg/day	[Delayed-release capsule 15, 30 mg]	L
Omeprazole (*Prilosec*)	20 mg qd x 8 weeks	60 mg/day	[Delayed-release capsule 10, 20 mg]	L

* Over-the-counter strength.

- Stop drugs that may promote reflux.
- Take medications with 6–8 oz. of water.
- Antacids.
- Surgery.

Helicobacter pylori is the major cause of peptic ulcer disease. Nonsteroidal anti-inflammatory drugs (NSAIDs) are the second most common cause.

Diagnosis of *H pylori*:
- Urea breath test.
- Serology.
- An endoscopic examination.

Initial treatment options:
- Empiric anti-ulcer treatment for 6 weeks.
- Definitive diagnostic evaluation by endoscopy.
- Noninvasive testing for *H pylori* and treatment with antibiotic for (+) patients (see **Tables 48** and **49**, p 105 for regimens).

Table 48. Oral Regimens for Treatment of H pylori

Bismuth Subsalicylate (B)	Tetracycline (T)	Metronidazole (M)	Clarithromycin (C)	Amoxicillin (A)	Omeprazole (O)	Ranitidine Bismuth Citrate (R)
2 tabs qid pc and hs	500 mg qid	250 mg qid pc and hs	500 mg qid or tid with meals	500 mg qid pc and hs	20 mg bid ac	400 mg bid

Regimens Using Oral Doses from Table 48

Combination (Duration)	Cure Rate, 95% CIs
BMT* (1 wk)	86–90
BMT* (2 wks)	88–90
BMT* and O (1 wk)	94–98
BMA (1 wk)	75–81

Combination (Duration)	Cure Rate, 95% CIs
BMA (2 wks)	80–86
BCT* (1–2 wks)	(>80%)
BCA (1–2 wks)	(>90%)
RC (2 wks)	82–94

*Separate bismuth and tetracycline by 2 hours.

Source: Adapted from Soll AH. Practice Parameters Committee of the American College of Gastroenterology. Medical treatment of peptic ulcer disease: Practice guidelines. JAMA. 1996;275:622–629. Copyright 1996– 97, American Medical Association. Reprinted with permission.

Table 49. Oral Regimens for H pylori

Omeprazole (O)	Lansoprazole (L)	Clarithromycin (C)	Amoxicillin (A)	Metronidazole (M)
20 mg bid ac and loading dose	30 mg bid	500 mg bid pc	1 g bid pc	500 mg bid pc

Regimens Using Oral Antibiotic Doses from Table 49

Combination (Duration)	Cure Rate, 95% CIs
MOC (1 wk)	87–91
AOC (1 wk)	86–91
MOA (1–2 wks)	77–83

Combination (Duration)	Cure Rate, 95% CIs
LCA (2 wks)	(94%)
LCM (1 wk)	(90%)

Source: Adapted from Soll AH. Practice Parameters Committee of the American College of Gastroenterology. Medical treatment of peptic ulcer disease: Practice guidelines. JAMA. 1996;275:622–629. Copyright 1996– 97, American Medical Association. Reprinted with permission.

Medications: Antibiotics (For complete information see "Infectious Diseases," p 78): Bismuth subsalicylate (*Pepto-Bismol*) [chewable tablet 262 mg; suspension 262 mg/15 mL]. Tetracycline (*Achromycin, Sumycin*) [tablet 250, 500 mg; suspension 125 mg/5 mL]. Metronidazole (*Flagyl*) [tablet 250, 500, 750 mg; capsule 375 mg]. Clarithromycin (*Biaxin*) [film-coated tablet 250, 500 mg; oral suspension 125 mg/5 mL, 250 mg/5 mL]. Amoxicillin (*Amoxil*) [capsule and chewable tablet 250, 500 mg; suspension 125 mg/5 mL, 250 mg/5 mL]. Proton-pump inhibitors: Omeprazole (*Prilosec*) [delayed-release capsule 10, 20 mg]. Lansoprazole (*Prevacid*) [delayed-release capsule 15, 30 mg]. H_2 antagonist combination: Ranitidine bismuth citrate [ranitidine 162 mg, trivalent bismuth 128 mg, and citrate 110 mg] (*Tritec*) [tablet 400 mg].

CONSTIPATION

Definition
Infrequent, incomplete, or painful evacuation of feces.

Drugs That Constipate
- Analgesics – opiates.
- Antacids with aluminum or calcium.
- Anticholinergic drugs.
- Antidepressants.
- Antihypertensives.
- Antipsychotics.
- Barium sulfate.
- Bismuth.
- Calcium channel blockers.
- Diuretics.
- Iron.

Conditions That Constipate
- Dehydration.
- Depression.
- Diabetes.
- Hypercalcemia.
- Hypokalemia.
- Hypothyroidism.
- Immobility.
- Panhypopituitarism.
- Parkinson's disease.
- Uremia.

Table 50 Drugs that May Relieve Constipation

Bulk-Producing Laxative	Onset of Action	Site of Action	Mechanism of Action	Recommended Starting Dose
Methylcellulose Psyllium (*Metamucil*)	12–24 h (up to 72 h)	Small and large intestine	Holds water in stool; mechanical distention	1–2 rounded tsp or packets qd–tid with water or juice
Malt soup extract (*Maltsupe*) Surfactants/Stool Softener		Surfactant/Stool Softener	Also, reduces fecal pH	Juice
Docusate (*Colace*) Saline	24–72 h	Small and large intestine	Detergent activity; facilitates admixture of fat and water to soften stool	100 mg qd–qid
Magnesium citrate (*Citroma*)	0.5–3 h	Small and large intestine	Attract/retain water in intestinal lumen	120–240 mL x 1
Magnesium hydroxide (*Milk of Magnesia*)				30 mL qd–bid
Sodium phosphate/biphosphate Emollient enema (*Fleets enema*)	2–15 min	Colon		One 4.5 oz. enema x 1, repeat prn
Sorbitol 70%	24–48 h	Colon	Delivers osmotically active molecules to colon	15–30 mL qd–bid
Lactulose (*Cephulac*)		Colon		15–30 mL qd–bid
Irritant/Stimulant Senna (*Senokot*)	6–10 h	Colon	Direct action on intestine; stimulate myenteric plexus; after water and electrolyte secretion	2 tabs or 1 tsp qhs
Bisacodyl Tab	0.25–1 h	Colon		Oral: 5–15 mg x 1
Bisacodyl Supp. (*Dulcolax*)				Supp. 10 mg x 1

ENDOCRINE DISORDERS

Corticosteroids/Adrenal Insufficiency
• Corticosteroids dose equivalency (see **Table 51**, p 109).
• Management: Stress doses of steroids for patients with severe illness, injury or undergoing surgery: Give hydrocortisone 100 mg IV q8h. For less severe stress, double or triple usual oral replacement dose and taper back to baseline as quickly as possible.

Thyroid Disease
• Pharmacologic therapy: Thyroxine (T_4, levothyroxine, [*Synthroid, Levoxyl*]). Start 25 μg and increase by 25 μg intervals of 25 μg every 4–6 weeks. For myxedema coma: Load 400 μg IV or 100 μg q6–8h for 1 day then 100 μg/day for 4 days; then start usual replacement regimen [25,50,75,88,100,112,125, 137,150,175,200,300 μg]. Iodine (*Thyro-Block*) 1 tab PO qd [130]. Liquid form: Lugol's Solution. Propylthiouracil (PTU): Start 100 PO tid, then adjust up to 200 PO tid as needed [50]. Methimazole (*Tapazole*): Start 5–20 mg PO tid, then adjust [5,10]. To convert thyroid USP to thyroxine: 60 mg USP = 50 μg thyroxine.
• Management/monitoring: In primary hypothyroidism, the goal of therapy is to maintain plasma TSH within the normal range. Because it may take several months for elevated plasma TSH to return to normal, it should be measured after 3–4 months of therapy. Further adjustments are made every 6–8 weeks (12–25 μg increments) based on TSH levels until TSH is in normal range. Monitor TSH level every 6–12 months (ATA) in patients on chronic thyroid replacement therapy. If patients are NPO and must receive IV thyroxine, dose should be half usual PO dose.

Diabetes
• Definition/classification (ADA): Diabetes mellitus is a group of metabolic diseases characterized by hyperglycemia resulting from defects in insulin secretion, insulin action, or both. Type 1 is caused by an absolute deficiency of insulin secretion. Type 2 is caused by a combination of resistance to insulin action and an inadequate compensatory insulin secretory response. Criteria for the diagnosis of diabetes include one or more of the following: (1) Symptoms of diabetes (eg, polyuria, polydipsia, unexplained weight loss) plus casual plasma glucose concentration ≥200 mg/dL; (2) Fasting (no caloric intake for ≥8h) plasma glucose ≥126 mg/dL; (3) 2h plasma glucose ≥200 mg/dL during an oral glucose tolerance test (OGTT). Diagnosis should be confirmed by reevaluating on a subsequent day. *Impaired fasting glucose* is defined as fasting plasma glucose ≥110 and <126 mg/dL. *Impaired glucose tolerance* is abnormal casual plasma glucose concentration or response to OGTT but not meeting diagnostic criteria for diabetes.
• Management (ADA): Goals of treatment: Fasting plasma glucose <120 mg/dL and Hb A_{1c} <7%.
  - **Nonpharmacologic interventions**: Individualized nutrition, lifestyle (eg, exercise, smoking cessation), patient and family education for self-management, self-monitoring of blood glucose.

Drug	Approximate Equivalent Dose (mg)	Relative Anti-inflammatory Potency	Relative Mineralocorticoid	Biologic Half-Life (hours)	How Supplied
Betamethasone (Celestone)	0.6–0.75	20–30	0	36–54	[6; 6 mg/5 mL]
Cortisone (Cortone)	25	0.8	2	8–12	[5; 50 mg/mL susp]
Dexamethasone (Decadron, Dexone, Hexadrol)	0.75	20–30	0	36–54	[.25, .5, .75, 1, 1.5, 2, 4; .5 mg/5 mL elixir; 4 mg/mL inj]
Hydrocortisone (Cortef)	20	1	2	8–12	[5, 10, 20; 50 mg/mL inj; 10 mg/5 mL susp]
Methylprednisolone (Medrol, SoluMedrol, Depo-Medrol)	4	5	0	18–36	[2, 4, 16, 24, 32, 40 mg, 125, 500, 1000 mg inj]
Prednisolone (Delta Cortef, Pretone Syrup, Pediapred)	5	4	1	18–36	[5, 15 mg/5 mL syrup; 5 mg/5 mL liquid]
Prednisone (Deltasone, LiquidPred, Orasone)	5	4	1	18–36	[1, 2.5, 5, 10, 20, 50; 5 mg/5 mL liquid]
Triamcinolone (Aristocort, Kenacort, Kenalog)	4	5	0	18–36	[1, 2, 4, 8; 4 mg/5 mL syrup]
Fludrocortisone (Florinef)*	N/A	10	4	12–36	[.1]

Table 51. Corticosteroids

*Usually given for orthostatic hypotension 0.1 mg 2–3 times/day.

Table 52. Oral Agents for Treating Diabetes

Drug	Dosage Ranges	How Supplied	Excretion	Comments
Sulfonylureas				
First Generation				
Acetohexamide – generic or (*Dymelor*)	250–1500 mg once or divided	[250, 500]	L,K	Long half-life of metabolite
Chlorpropamide – generic or (*Diabinese*)	125–500 mg once	[100, 250]	L,K	Long-acting, risk of hypoglycemia and hyponatremia
Tolazamide – generic or (*Tolinase, Ronase*)	100–1000 mg once or divided	[100, 250, 500]	L,K	
Tolbutamide – generic or (*Orinase*)	250–3000 mg once or divided	[500]	L,K	Numerous drug interactions
Second Generation				
Glimepiride (*Amaryl*)	4–8 mg once, begin 1–2 mg	[1, 2, 4]	L,K	Numerous drug interactions, long-acting
Glipizide – generic or (*Glucotrol*)	2.5–20 mg once or divided	[5, 10]	L,K	
(*Glucotrol XL*) sustained-release tablets	5–10 mg once	[5, 10]	L,K	Long-acting
Glyburide – generic or (*DiaBeta, Micronase*)	1.25–20 mg once or divided	[1.25, 2.5, 5]	L,K	Long-acting, risk of hypoglycemia
Micronized glyburide (*Glynase*)	1.5–12 mg once	[1.5, 3, 6]	L,K	
Alpha-glucosidase inhibitor				
Acarbose (*Precose*)	50–100 mg tid, just before meals, start with 25 mg	[50, 100]	gut/K	GI side effects are common, avoid if Cr >2 mg/dL, monitor LFTs
Biguanide				
Metformin (*Glucophage*)	500–2550, divided	[500, 850]	K	Avoid in patients ≥ 80 years, renal insufficiency, CHF, COPD, if increased LFTs, avoid IV contrast agents
Benzoic Acid Derivative				
Repaglinide (*Prandin*)	0.5–4 times/day if Hb A1c < 8% or previously untreated. 1–2 mg 2–4 times/day if Hb A1c ≥ 8% or previously treated	[0.5, 1, 2]	L	Give 30 minutes before meals, adjust dose at weekly intervals, potential for drug interactions, caution in liver or renal insufficiency
Thiazolidinedione				
Troglitazone (*Rezulin*)	200–500 mg once	[200, 300, 400]	L	Check LFTs at start, then monthly for 8 months, then periodically q 2 months for 4 months, then periodically

Insulin Preparations	Onset	Peak	Duration
Insulin lispro (*Humalog*)	5–30 min	1–2 h	2–4 h
Insulin (*Iletin, Novolin, Humulin*)			
Regular	1/2–1 h	2–4 h	4–6 h
NPH	2–4 h	8–12 h	24 h
(also available as mixtures of NPH/regular in 70:30 and 50:50 proportions)			
Ultralente	4–8 h	10–30 h	>36 h

- **Pharmacologic interventions for Type 2 diabetes**: Stepped therapy: (1) Monotherapy with sulfonylurea agent, acarbose, troglitazone, or metformin; (2) combination therapy with 2 or more agents; (3) add or switch to insulin (see **Table 52** and p 111).
- **Monitoring (ADA)**: Weight, blood pressure, and foot examination each visit. Hb A$_{1c}$ once or twice a year in patients with stable glycemic control; quarterly in patients who are in poor control. Annual comprehensive dilated eye and visual examinations by an ophthalmologist or optometrist who is knowledgeable and experienced in the management of diabetic retinopathy. Lipid profiles every 1–5 years depending on whether values are in normal range. Annual urinalysis. If the urinalysis is negative for protein, test for microalbuminuria by measuring albumin to creatinine ratio in a random spot collection, timed collection, or 24-hr collection.

WOMEN'S HEALTH

Prevention
Annual breast and pelvic/perineal examination; one negative pap smear after 65 years, if low risk (ie, single established sexual partner); annual mammography as appropriate; osteoporosis evaluation (see "Osteoporosis," p 36). Discuss hormone replacement therapy.

Common disorders
• Vulvar diseases:
- **Nonneoplastic:** Lichen sclerosus – occurs anywhere on the body at any age, but is most common on vulva of middle-aged and older women; causes 1/3 of benign vulvar lesions, extends to perirectal areas (classic hour glass appearance); lesions are white to pink macules or papules, may coalesce; symptoms are none or itching, soreness, or dyspareunia. Must biopsy for diagnosis. Treatment: Petrolatum or testosterone propionate 2% or clobetasol propionate 0.05% daily for 12 weeks, then prn.
- **Squamous hyperplasia:** Raised white keratinized lesions difficult to distinguish from vulvar intraepithelial neoplasia (VIN); must biopsy to exclude malignancy; topical steroids bid until lesions resolve.
- **Neoplastic:** VIN – most often seen in postmenopausal women; asymptomatic or may cause pruritus; appear as white keratinized lesions; often

multifocal; colposcopy of the entire vulva with biopsy is necessary; lesions graded on degree of atypia; treatment is surgical or other ablative therapy.

- **Vulvar malignancy:** Highly age-related; half of cases occur >70 years; 80% are squamous cell, with melanoma, sarcoma, basal cell, and adenocarcinoma <20%; biopsy any suspicious lesion; radical surgery is preferred treatment.

• Other

- Postmenopausal bleeding: Bleeding after 1 year of amenorrhea is common; evaluation and treatment aim at excluding malignancy, treating symptoms and identifying cause; examine genitalia, perineum, rectum; for endometrial source either endometrial biopsy or vaginal probe ultrasound to assess endometrial thickness (<5 mm virtually excludes malignancy); dilation and curettage (D&C) when endometrium not otherwise adequately assessed. Women on combination continuous estrogen and progesterone who bleed after 12 months need evaluation; those on cyclic replacement with bleeding at unexpected times need evaluation.

- Hot flushes: Vasomotor symptoms respond to estrogen (see **Table 53**, p 113) in dose response fashion; start low dose, titrate to effect. If estrogen cannot be taken, less effective alternatives: megestrol (*Megace*): [20, 40 mg] 20 mg bid; medroxyprogesterone acetate (*Provera Cycerin*): [2.5, 5, 10 mg] or clonidine (*Catapres*): [0.1, 0.2, 0.3 mg] 0.1-0.3 mg/day may be tried.

- Vaginal prolapse: Child-bearing and other causes of increased intra-abdominal pressure weaken connective tissue and muscles supporting the genital organs leading to prolapse. Symptoms include: Pelvic pressure, back pain, fecal or urinary incontinence, or difficulty evacuating the rectum. The degree of prolapse and organs involved dictate therapy; no therapy if asymptomatic. Estrogen and Kegel's exercises may help in mild cases. Pessary or surgery indicated with greater symptoms. Precise anatomic defect(s) dictates the surgical approach. Symptoms may be present even with mild prolapse. A common (ACOG) classification for degrees of prolapse: First degree - extension to the mid vagina; second degree - approaching the hymenal ring; third degree - at the hymenal ring; and fourth degree - beyond the hymenal ring.

- Atrophic vaginitis (see "Sexual Dysfunction," p 114).

Hormone Replacement Therapy

• Estrogen replacement after menopause has been associated with preservation of bone mass, lowered cardiovascular risk, and perhaps maintaining cognitive capacity. Positive effects on urogenital health include reduced dyspareunia and maintaining continence. When the patient has a uterus, estrogen should be combined with progesterone to reduce endometrial cancer. Some women prefer unopposed estrogen and annual biopsy. Common dose regimens are given in **Table 53**, p 113).

• Estrogen risks/side effects: Estrogen therapy increases risk of endometrial cancer, but the effect is attenuated or eliminated by progestational agents; breast cancer risk probably increased by higher dose and with long-term use.

- Contraindications to estrogen: Undiagnosed vaginal bleeding, active thromboembolic disease, probably breast cancer, endometrial cancer greater than stage 1, possibly gall bladder disease, menstrual migraine.

Table 53. Common Regimens for Hormone Replacement Therapy				
Preparation	Dose	Cyclic Dosing	Continuous Dosing	Formulations
Conjugated equine estrogen (Premarin)	0.3–0.625 mg/d	Days 1–25	Daily	[0.3, 0.625, 0.9, 1.25, 2.5]
Micronized 17-beta estradiol (Estrace)	0.5–1.0 mg/d	Days 1–25	Daily	[.5, 1, 2]
Transdermal estrogen (Estraderm, Vivelle, Climara, Alora)	0.025–0.1 mg patches	Biweekly for 3 weeks, then 1 week off	Biweekly	Alora [0.5, 0.75, 1]; Estraderm, Climara [0.05]; Vivelle [0.0375, 0.05, 0.075, 0.1]
Fempatch	.025 mg/d	Weekly for 3 weeks, 1 week off	Weekly	[0.025]
Medroxyprogesterone (Cycrin, Provera)	2.5–10.0 mg/d	5–10 mg days 1–14	2.5–5.0 mg daily	[2.5, 5, 10]
Combination Drugs				
Conjugated estrogen + medroxyprogesterone (Prempro)	0.625 mg 2.5 mg	N/A	Daily	Fixed dose
Conjugated estrogen + medroxyprogesterone (Premphase)	0.625 mg 5.0 mg	Days 1–28 Days 14–28	N/A	Fixed dose

113

SEXUAL DYSFUNCTION

IMPOTENCE (ERECTILE DYSFUNCTION)

Definition: Inability to achieve erection sufficient for intercourse, prevalence nearly 70% by age 70.

Causes: >50% of cases arterial, venous or mixed vascular cause; other causes include drug side effects, thyroid or adrenal disorders, hyperprolactinemia, hypogonadism, diabetes, disorders of the CNS, spinal cord, or PNS, autonomic neuropathy, temporal lobe epilepsy, depression, anxiety, bereavement. Decreased bioavailable testosterone is more associated with decreased libido than erectile dysfunction. Erectile dysfunction is often multifactorial.

Evaluation:

- History: Type and duration of problem; relation to surgery, trauma, medication. Problems with orgasm, libido, or penile detumescence are not erectile dysfunction.
- Physical Characteristics: Look for orthostatic hypotension, impaired response to Valsalva maneuver, absent bulbocavernosus or cremasteric reflexes suggest neuropathy; penile bands, plaques suggest Peyronie's disease; diminished male pattern hair, gynecomastia, small (<20–25 mm long) testes suggest hypogonadism.
- Assessment:
  - Reduced penile to brachial pressure index suggests vascular disease.
  - Cavernosometry diagnoses venous leak syndrome; reserved for surgical candidates.
  - Test dose of prostaglandin E or papaverine can exclude vascular disease or confirm venous leak syndrome.
  - For libido problems check total and bioavailable testosterone, LH, TSH, and prolactin.

Therapy: Sildenafil (Viagra [25, 50, 100 mg]) has been studied for erectile dysfunction of various etiologies (organic, psychogenic, mixed); vascular impotence is least likely to respond; contraindicated with use of nitrates. Several other important drug interactions; metabolism reduced in liver disease, kidney disease, and aging. Starting dose 25 mg 1hr before sexual activity. Use maximum once daily. Side effects: headache, flushing, dyspepsia, mild and transient, predominantly color tinge in vision, nasal congestion, urinary tract infection, diarrhea, dizziness, and rash.

DYSPAREUNIA

Definition

Pain with intercourse.

Aggravating factors: Vaginal atrophy from estrogen deprivation, vulvar or vaginal infection, interstitial cystitis, retroverted uterus, gynecologic tumors, osteoarthritis, sacral nerve root compression, pelvic fractures, myalgia from overexertion during Kegel's exercises.

Evaluation: Physician should make patient feel comfortable and ask about sexual problems; (eg, changes in libido, partner's function, and health issues); screen for depression. Pelvic examination for vulvovaginitis, vaginal atrophy, conization (decreased distensibility and narrowing of the vaginal canal), scarring, pelvic inflammatory disease, cystocele, and rectocele.

Management: Identify and treat clinical pathology; educate and counsel patients; discuss hormone replacement therapy (see "Women's Health," p 111). For atrophic vaginitis, topical estrogens (see "Women's Health," p 111); water-soluble lubricants (*Replens*) are highly effective as monotherapy for those who cannot or will not use hormones, or as a supplement to estrogen. For vaginismus (vaginal muscle spasm), trial cessation of intercourse and gradual vaginal dilation. For diminished libido, short-term androgens (which long-term adversely affect health) may help; refer for counseling or sex therapy. Topical estrogens (*Premarin* [0.625 g], *Ogen* [0.625, 1.25, 2.0], *Orthodienestorol, Estrace* [0.5, 1, 2]), use miminum dose (eg, 0.5 g *Premarin*, 2 g *Ogen* or *Estrace*) daily for 2 weeks, then 1–3 times a week thereafter; controls symptoms. Estradriol vaginal ring (*Estring*) inserted intravaginally and changed every 90 days.

Table 54. Management of Erectile Dysfunction		
Cause	Therapy	Side Effects/ Acceptability/Cautions
Poor libido/hypogonadism	Testosterone scrotal transdermal (*Testoderm*) [4, 6] 4–6 mg qd; or skin transdermal (*Androderm*) [2.5, 5] 5 mg/day; or testosterone cypionate or enanthate 200 mg IM q 2–4 weeks	When given, IM can cause polycythemia, potential for increased prostate size, fluid retention, gynecomastia, liver dysfunction
Vascular/neuropathic/or mixed	Vacuum tumescence devices	Rare: Ecchymosis, reduced ejaculation, coolness of penile tip. Good acceptance in older population; intercourse successful 70% to 90% cases
	Intracavernosal [5, 10, 20, 40 µg] or intraurethral [250, 500] prostaglandin E (*Alprostadil*)	Risks: Hypotension, bruising, bleeding, priapism; erection >4 hr requires emergency treatment; intraurethral safer and more acceptable
	Penile prosthesis	Complications: Infection, mechanical failure, penile fibrosis

HEMATOLOGY/ONCOLOGY

Evaluation and Treatment of Anemia

Overview: Some decrease in hemoglobin with age; after age 65 evaluate when Hb < 12 in men and when <11.5 in women; evaluate if Hb falls > 1 g/dL in 1 year; evaluate when evidence of bleeding.

Evaluation: Check reticulocyte and cell size and evaluate for hypo- or hyper-regenerative disorder; bone marrow aspirate and biopsy if etiology not clear. The evaluation and management of hyporegenerative anemia is given in

Table 55, p 117. Myelodysplastic anemias, a clonal disorder with macrocytic red cells, and abnormal red cell precursors in bone marrow; five subtypes which determine outcome; primary treatment is supportive with blood component transfusions, erythropoietin may help; other therapy depends on subtype. An overview of the more common forms of hyperregenerative anemias is given in **Table 56**, p 117.

Many older individuals receive long-term drug therapy for cancers of the breast and prostate. The uses and side effects of the agents are reviewed here.

Cancer
Breast Cancer
- Monitoring: History, physical, LFTs, calcium every 4–6 months for 5 years, then yearly, annual mammography, pelvic, and stool for occult blood. Consider endometrial biopsy or vaginal probe ultrasound monitoring if patient is on tamoxifen.
- Pharmacotherapy
  – Postmenopausal women with estrogen receptor (ER) or progesterone receptor (PR) positive tumors who are at high risk for recurrence (tumors greater than 1 cm, or positive nodes) should be treated with tamoxifen (*Nolvadex*) 20 mg po qd [10, 20] for 5 years. Tamoxifen is hepatically metabolized; metabolism inhibited by erythromycin, cyclosporin, nifedipine, and diltiazem. Under 10% renally excreted, no dose reduction necessary in mild to moderate renal impairment; some increased risk of endometrial cancer, annual pelvic examination needed; annual eye examination also for possible retinitis; some increased risk of clotting, use with caution in women with clotting history. Women who fail tamoxifen and who are not chemotherapy candidates can be treated with anastrozole (*Arimidex*) 1 mg po qd [1] liver metabolism.
  – Adjuvant chemotherapy reduces recurrence risk for receptor-negative tumors. Combination chemotherapy with cyclophosphamide, methotrexate, fluorouracil or doxorubicin-containing regimens are beneficial. There is an additional 5%–10% reduction in recurrence in ER- or PR-positive tumors treated with both tamoxifen and chemotherapy.

Prostate Cancer Pharmacotherapy
- Hormonal therapy is indicated in locally advanced ≥ stage III or T3 (tumor extension beyond the prostate capsule) and metastatic prostate cancer. Drugs of choice are leuprolide or goserelin with or without flutamide. Other alternatives are also listed below.
- LH-RH agonists leuprolide acetate (*Lupron Depot*) [7.5 mg IM q month; or 22.5 mg q 3 months; or 30 mg q 4 months]; no pharmacokinetic studies are available; certain symptoms (obstruction, spinal cord compression, bone pain) may be exacerbated early in treatment; side effects—hot flushes (60%), edema (12%), pain (7%), nausea, vomiting, impotence, dyspnea, asthenia (all 5%).
- Goserelin acetate implant (*Zoladex*) [3.6 mg sc q 28 days or 10.8 mg q 3 months]; rapid urinary hepatic excretion, no dose adjustment in renal impairment; side effects—hot flushes (60%), breast swelling, libido change, impotence.

Table 55. The Diagnosis and Management of Hyporegenerative Anemia

Anemia Type	Diagnostic Findings and Considerations	Management
Chronic disorders	Chronic underlying disease Normocytic or microcytic RBCs Absent sideroblasts in marrow Differential diagnosis: Iron deficiency; sideroblastic anemia; heavy metal intoxication; thalassemia minor	Treat underlying disorder Erythropoietin 50–100 U/kg 3 x/wk; increase dose to 150 U/kg if no response in 2–3 weeks
Iron deficiency	Absent bone marrow hemosiderin Serum ferritin ≤ 50 µg/L with transferrin saturation ≤.08 Serum ferritin ≤20 µg/L Dietary history; stool for occult blood; blood smear for microcytosis, hypochromasia; GI evaluation	Correct cause of blood loss Oral iron supplements; parenteral iron if iron absorption poor
B$_{12}$ deficiency	Smear for macrocytosis, giant and multilobar neutrophils, decreased platelets; Serum B$_{12}$, folate, and TSH; methylmalonic and homocysteine in selected patients Schilling test	B$_{12}$, 1000 µg/week for 5 weeks; then 100 µg/month for life Potassium for the first week and iron supplement if anemia is severe
Aplastic anemia	Pancytopenia Bone marrow aspirate and biopsy Rule out hairy cell leukemia with tartrate resistant-acid phosphatase Rule out myelodysplastic syndrome with bone marrow and chromosomes	Cyclosporine Antithymocytic immunoglobulin

Source: Modified from *Geriatric Review Syllabus III*. Reprinted with permission.

Table 56. Diagnosis and Management of Hyperregenerative Anemia

Anemia Type	Diagnostic Findings and Considerations	Management
Autoimmune hemolytic anemia	Microspherocytes, cold and warm agglutinating antibodies Differential diagnosis: Lymphocytic lymphoma, chronic lymphocytic leukemia, collagen vascular disease, infection, medication-induced idiopathic	Warm agglutinating antibodies: Prednisone 100 mg/daily, and cyclophosphamide, or splenectomy; IV immunoglobulins [.4 g/kg/ day for 5 days] for life-threatening disease Cold agglutinating antibodies: Avoid cold temperatures; plasmapheresis; RBC transfusion during hemolysis may be hazardous
Microangiopathic hemolytic anemia	Circulating schistocytes, hemoglobinuria, hemosiderinuria Differential diagnosis: diabetes, atherosclerosis, collagen vascular disease Acute forms: hypertensive crisis, vasculitis, disseminated intravascular coagulation, thrombotic thrombocytopenic purpura (TTP)	Iron and folate replacement; autoimmune TTP- prednisone [60 mg/day for 2–3 weeks, then taper] or plasmapheresis

Antiandrogens

- Flutamide (*Eulexin*) [125] 125 mg caps 2 po q 8 hr; renally excreted; side effects—gynecomastia and/or galactorrhea (42%), diarrhea, nausea, vomiting, transaminase elevation.
- Nilutamide (*Nilandron*) [50] 300 mg for 30 days, then 150 mg po qd; liver metabolism, renal excretion; side effects—gynecomastia, nausea, vomiting, transaminase elevation, delayed light adaptation (90%), alcohol intolerance.
- Bicalutamide (*Casodex*) [50] 50 mg po qd; metabolized in liver, excreted in urine; half-life 10 days at steady state; side effects—hot flushes, breast pain, gynecomastia, hematuria, diarrhea, liver enzyme elevations.
- Ketoconazole (*Nizoral*) [200] 400 mg po q 8 hrs; half-life biphasic 2 hrs, 8 hrs; liver metabolism, bile excretion; side effects—hypoadrenalism, hypothyroidism, blood dyscrasias, fatigue, confusion, gynecomastia, hepatitis. There are numerous drug interactions.
- Estramustine phosphate sodium (estradiol linked to nitrogen mustard) (*Emcyt*) [140 mg] 10–16 mg/kg/day, on empty stomach; metabolized to estrogen analogues; contraindications—active thromboembolic disorders, use with caution in liver disease; side effects—fluid retention, glucose intolerance, hypertension, nausea, diarrhea, gynecomastia, transaminase elevation.
- Cyproterone acetate (*Androcur*) [50] 100 mg po bid-tid; liver metabolism, excreted in urine and feces; side effects—impotence, hepatotoxicity; cardiovascular side effects—edema, thromboembolism, MI, stroke but less than with DES.

RENAL AND PROSTATE DISORDERS

ACUTE RENAL FAILURE

Definition: An acute deterioration in renal function defined by decreased urine output and/or increased values of renal function tests.

Evaluation
Review medication list, bladder catheterization with determination of postvoid residual, urinalysis, renal ultrasonography, fractional excretion of sodium (Na)

$$\text{Fractional excretion of sodium} = \frac{\text{urine Na/plasma Na} \times 100\%}{\text{urine creatinine/plasma creatinine}}$$

[Prerenal < 1%, renal (ATN) > 1%]

Precipitating and Aggravating Factors
Volume depletion, acute tubular necrosis due to hypoperfusion and nephrotoxins, medications (eg, aminoglycosides, radiocontrast materials, nonsteroidal anti-inflammatory agents, and angiotensin-converting enzyme inhibitors).

Causes of Hyponatremia

- With increased plasma osmolality: Hyperglycemia (1.6 mEq/L decrement for each 100 mg/dL increase in plasma glucose);
- With normal plasma osmolality (pseudohyponatremia): Severe hyperlipidemia, hyperproteinemia (eg, multiple myeloma);
- With decreased plasma osmolality:
  - With extracellular fluid (ECF) excess: Renal failure (urine Na >20 mEq/L), heart failure, hepatic cirrhosis, nephrotic syndrome (urine Na <20 mEq/L but may be higher if using diuretics).
  - With decreased ECF volume: Renal losses from salt-losing nephropathies, diuretics, osmotic diuresis (urine Na >20 mEq/L); extrarenal loss due to vomiting, diarrhea, skin losses, and third-spacing (usually urine Na <20 mEq/L).
  - With normal ECF volume: Primary polydipsia; thiazide diuretics; hypothyroidism; adrenal insufficiency; SIADH due to drugs (eg, SSRI antidepressants, chlorpropamide), pulmonary disease, carcinoma.

Benign Prostatic Hyperplasia (BPH)

- Evaluation (AHCPR guidelines): Detailed medical history focusing on the urinary tract; physical examination including a digital rectal examination and a focused neurologic examination; urinalysis; measurement of serum creatinine. Measurement of prostatic specific antigen is optional.
- Medical treatment:
  - Alpha blockers: Terazosin (*Hytrin*) advance as tolerated—days 1 to 3, 1 mg/day at bedtime; days 4 to 7, 2 mg; days 8 to 14, 5 mg; day 15 and beyond 10 mg [1,2,5,10]. Doxazosin (*Cardura*) start 0.5 mg with maximum of 16 mg/day [1,2,4,8]. Prazosin (*Minipress*) start 1 mg/day (first dose at bedtime) or bid with maximum 20 mg/day [1,2,5]. Tamsulosin (*Flowmax*) 0.4 mg 1/2 hour after the same meal each day and increase to 0.8 mg if no response in 2-4 weeks [0.4].
  - 5-alpha reductase inhibitors: Finasteride (*Proscar*) 5 mg/day [5].
- Surgical management (AHCPR guidelines): Indicated if recurrent urinary tract infection, recurrent or persistent gross hematuria, bladder stones, or renal insufficiency are clearly secondary to BPH or as indicated by symptoms, patient preference, or failure of medical treatment. Options are: Transurethral resection of the prostate (TURP); transurethral incision of the prostate (TUIP), which is limited to prostates whose estimated resected tissue weight would be 30 grams or less; open prostatectomy for large glands.

COMMON DERMATOLOGIC CONDITIONS

Table 57. Dermatologic Conditions Described

Condition	Areas Affected	Description	Factors	Treatment
Xerosis (dry skin)	All skin surfaces	Dull, rough, flaky, cracked; nummular eczema	Low humidity, winter, aging	Thumidity, apply emollient ointment immediately after bathing; oatmeal baths; hydrocortisone 1% ointment; avoid excess bathing and bath oils (falls)
Neurodermatitis	Any skin surfaces	Generalized/localized itching	Irritants, xerosis, scabies, allergic contact dermatitis	Topical corticosteroids; rule out other causes
Seborrheic dermatitis	Nasal labial folds, eyebrows, hairline, side burns, posterior auriculare and mid-chest	Greasy, yellow scales with or without erythematous base; common in Parkinson's disease	All age groups	Hydrocortisone 1% cream bid or triamcinolone 0.1% ointment bid x 2 weeks; scalp - shampoo (selenium sulfide, zinc or tar)
Rosacea	Face	Vascular and follicular dilation; mild to moderate		Topical metronidazole gel 0.75% bid Oral doxycycline 100mg qd
Onychomycosis	Nails	Thickening and discoloration of nails		Itraconazole (Sporanox) 200 mg po qd x 3 months (toenails), L; Terbinafine (Lamisil) 250 mg po qd x 6 wks (fingernails), 12 weeks (toenails)
Psoriasis	All skin areas, nails (pitting)	Well-defined, erythematous plaques covered with silver scales; severity varies	All ages, can be drug-induced	Topical corticosteroids, UV light, PUVA, methotrexate, cyclosporin, etretinate, sulfasalazine
Intertrigo	Any place where 2 skin surfaces rest against one another, leg, under the breasts)	Moist, erythematous with local superficial skin loss. Satellite lesions due to candida.	Obesity, diabetes melitus, immobility	Keep the area dry; topical antifungals (see p 122), absorbent powder; 1% hydrocortisone cream if inflamed

Table 57. Dermatologic Conditions Described (cont.)

Condition	Areas Affected	Description	Factors	Treatment
Candidiasis	Body folds	Erythema, pustules or cheesy, whitish matter, satellite lesions	Intertrigo, diabetes, poor hygiene	See intertrigo, antifungal powders
Scabies	Interdigital webs, flexor aspects of wrists, axillary, umbilicus, nipples, genitalia	Burrows, erythematous papules or nodules, dry or scaly skin, pruritus	Can result in epidemics	Topical 5% permethrin cream or 1% lindane cream left on overnight. Re-treat in 7 days. Oatmeal baths, topical corticosteroids or emollient creams for symptom relief

TREATMENT

Medications

Topical Corticosteroids
- Lowest potency: Hydrocortisone acetate (*Hytone*) [1%, 2.5%]; dexamethasone phosphate (*Decaderm*).
- Low potency: Alclometasone dipropionate [0.05% ointment or cream] (*Aclovate*); triamcinolone acetonide [0.1% cream] (*Aristocort, Kenalog*); fluocinolone acetonide [0.025% cream, 0.01% solution] (*Synalar*); betamethasone valerate [0.1% lotion] (*Valisone*); desonide [0.05% cream] (*DesOwen, Tridesilon*).
- Midpotency: Flurandrenolide [0.05% cream or ointment] (*Cordran*); fluticasone propionate [0.05% cream] (*Cutivate*); betamethasone dipropionate [0.05% lotion] (*Diprosone*); triamcinolone acetonide [0.1% lotion] (*Aristocort, Kenalog*); hydrocortisone butyrate [0.1% cream] (*Locoid*); fluocinolone acetonide [0.025% cream or ointment] (*Synalar*); betamethasone valerate [0.1% cream] (*Valisone*); hydrocortisone valerate [0.2% cream or ointment] (*Westcort*); triamcinolone acetonide [0.1% ointment] (*Aristocort, Kenalog*); mometasone furoate [0.1% cream] (*Elocon*).
- High potency: Triamcinolone acetonide [0.5% ointment] (*Aristocort, Kenalog*); fluticasone propionate [0.005% ointment] (*Cutivate*); amcinonide [0.1% cream, 0.1% lotion] (*Cyclocort*); betamethasone dipropionate [0.05% cream] (*Diprosone, Maxivate*); diflorasone diacetate [0.05% cream] (*Florone, Maxiflor*); fluocinonide [0.05% cream] (*Lidex-E*); betamethasone valerate [0.01% ointment] (*Valisone*).
- Higher potency: Amcinonide [0.1% ointment] (*Cyclocort*); betamethasone dipropionate [0.05% (optimized) cream] (*Diprolene AF*); betamethasone dipropionate [0.05% ointment] (*Diprosone, Maxivate*); mometasone furoate [0.1% ointment] (*Elocon*); diflorasone diacetate [0.05% ointment] (*Florone, Maxiflor*); halcinonide [0.1% cream] (*Halog*); fluocinonide [0.05% ointment, 0.05% cream, 0.05% gel] (*Lidex*); desoximetasone [0.05% gel, 0.25% cream, 0.25% ointment] (*Topicort*).
- Super potency: Clobetasol propionate [0.05% cream and ointment] (*Temovate*); betamethasone dipropionate [0.05% cream and ointment] (*Diprolene*); halobetasol propionate [0.05% cream and ointment] (*Ultravate*); diflorasone diacetate [0.05% (optimized) ointment] (*Psorcon*).

Topical antifungals
- Amphotericin B [3% cream, lotion, or ointment] (*Fungizone*); clotrimazole [1% cream, lotion, solution] (*Lotrimin, Mycelex*); econazole nitrate [1% cream] (*Spectazole*); ketoconazole [2% cream or shampoo] (*Nizoral*); miconazole [2% cream, lotion, powder, spray, tincture] (*Monistat-Derm, others*); nystatin [100,000 units/g cream, ointment, powder] (*Mycostatin, Nilstat, Nystex*).

Scabicides
- Permethrin [5% cream, 1% creme rinse] (*Elimite*); lindane [1% cream, lotion, shampoo] (*K-well, Scabene*); crotamiton [10% cream, lotion] (*Eurax*).

MISCELLANEOUS MEDICATIONS

Antiplatelet Agents

Aspirin: 81–325 mg po daily [T: 81, 325, 500 mg; CT: 81 mg; Suppository: 120, 200, 300, 600, mg].

Clopidogrel (*Plavix*): 75 mg po qd [T: 75 mg].

Ticlopidine (*Ticlid*): 250 mg po bid with food. Monitor CBC with differential (for agranulocytosis and anemia) q2 weeks through the first 3 months [T: 250 mg].

Nicotine for Smoking Cessation

Transdermal patch (patients should be advised to completely stop smoking upon initiation of therapy): Apply new patch q24h to nonhairy, clean, dry skin on the upper body or upper outer arm; each patch should be applied to a different site.

• Initial starting dosage: 21 mg/day for 4-8 weeks for most patients.

• First weaning dosage: 14 mg/day for 2-4 weeks.

• Second weaning dosage: 7 mg/day for 2-4 weeks.

Initial starting dosage for patients <100 lbs, who smoke <10 cigarettes/day, have a history of cardiovascular disease: 14 mg/day for 4-8 weeks followed by 7 mg/day for 2-4 weeks.

In patients who are receiving >600 mg/day of cimetidine: Decrease to the next lower patch size.

Metabolism is through the liver.

Transdermal patches available over the counter:

Habitrol: 21 mg/day; 14 mg/day; 7 mg/day [30 systems/box]
Nicoderm: 21 mg/day; 14 mg/day; 7 mg/day [14 systems/box]
Nicotrol: 15 mg/day (gradually released over 16 hours)
Prostep: 22 mg/day; 11 mg/day [7 systems/box]

Gum: Chew 1 piece when urge to smoke, up to 30 pieces/day; most patients require 10-12 pieces of gum/day.

Pieces, chewing gum, as polacrilex: 2 mg/square (OTC) [96 pieces/box]; 4 mg/square [96 pieces/box].

Antiemetics

Buclizine (*Bucladin-S*) Softab: [Tablet, chewable, 50 mg]. Motion sickness (prophylaxis): 50 mg 30 minutes prior to traveling; may repeat 50 mg after 4-6 hours. Vertigo: 50 mg twice daily, up to 150 mg/day.

Chlorpromazine (*Thorazine*): [Capsule, sustained action: 30, 75, 150, 200, 300 mg; concentrate, oral: 30; 100 mg/mL; injection: 25 mg/mL; suppository, rectal: 25, 100 mg; syrup: 10 mg/5 mL; tablet: 10, 25, 50, 100, 200 mg]. Oral: 10-25 mg q4-6h; IM, IV: 25-50 mg q4-6h; rectal: 50-100 mg q6-8h. L.

Cisapride (*Propulsid*): [Suspension, oral: 1 mg/mL; tablet, scored: 10, 20 mg]. Initial: 10 mg qid 15 minutes ac and hs; in some patients the dosage will need to be increased to 20 mg. L.

Cyclizine (*Marezine*): [Injection, as lactate: 50 mg/mL; tablet: 50 mg]. Oral: 25-50 mg taken 30 minutes before departure, may repeat in 4-6 hours if needed, up to 200 mg/day; IM: 25-50 mg q4-6h as needed.

Dexamethasone (*Decadron*): [Solution, oral: Concentrate: 0.5 mg/0.5 mL (30% alcohol); oral: 0.5 mg/5 mL; tablet: 0.25, 0.5, 0.75, 1, 1.5, 2, 4, 6 mg; injection, as acetate suspension: 8,16 mg/mL; injection, as sodium phosphate: 4, 10, 20, 24 mg/mL]. Oral/IV (should be given as sodium phosphate): 10 mg/m^2/dose (usually 20 mg) for first dose then 5 mg/m^2/dose q6h as needed. L.

Dimenhydrinate (*Dramamine*): [Capsule: 50 mg; injection: 50 mg/mL; liquid: 12.5 mg/4 mL, 16.62 mg/5 mL; tablet: 50 mg; tablet, chewable: 50 mg]. Oral, IM, IV: 50-100 mg q4-6h, not to exceed 400 mg/day. L.

Dronabinol (*Marinol*): [Capsule: 2.5, 5, 10 mg]. 5 mg/m^2 1-3 hours before chemotherapy, then administer 5 mg/m^2/dose q2-4h after chemotherapy for a total of 4-6 doses/day; dose may be increased up to a maximum of 15 mg/m^2/dose if needed (dosage may be increased by 2.5-mg/m^2 increments). L.

Droperidol (*Inapsine*): [Injection: 2.5 mg/mL]. Premedication IM: 2.5-10 mg 30 minutes to 1 hour preoperatively. Adjunct to general anesthesia: IV induction: 0.22-0.275 mg/kg; maintenance: 1.25-2.5 mg/dose; alone in diagnostic procedures: IM: Initial: 2.5-10 mg 30 minutes to 1 hour before; then 1.25-2.5 mg if needed; nausea and vomiting: IM, IV: 2.5-5 mg/dose q3-4h as needed. L/R.

Granisetron (*Kytril*): [Injection: 1 mg/mL; tablet: 1 mg]. IV: 10 μg/kg for 1-3 doses; oral: Adults: 1 mg twice daily; the first 1-mg dose should be given up to 1 hour before chemotherapy, and the second tablet 12 hours after the first. L.

Meclizine (*Antivert*): [Capsule: 15, 25, 30 mg; tablet: 12.5, 25, 50 mg, chewable: 25 mg; film coated: 25 mg]. Motion sickness: 12.5-25 mg 1 hour before travel, repeat dose q12-24h if needed; doses up to 50 mg may be needed; vertigo: 25-100 mg/day in divided doses. L.

Metoclopramide (*Reglan*): [Injection: 5 mg/mL; solution, oral, concentrated: 10 mg/mL; syrup, sugar free: 5 mg/5 mL; tablet: 5, 10 mg]. Chemotherapy-induced emesis: IV: 1-2 mg/kg 30 minutes before chemotherapy and q2-4h to q4-6h; postoperative nausea and vomiting: IM: 5-10 mg near end of surgery. R.

Ondansetron (*Zofran*): [Injection: 2 mg/mL, 32 mg (single-dose vials); tablet: 4, 8 mg >80 kg: 12 mg IVPB; 45-80 kg: 8 mg IVPB; <45 kg: 0.15 mg/kg/dose IVPB]. Maximum daily dose: 8 mg in cirrhotic patients with severe liver disease. L.

Perphenazine (*Trilafon*): [Concentrate, oral: 16 mg/5 mL; injection: 5 mg/mL; tablet: 2, 4, 8, 16 mg]. Oral: 8-16 mg/day in divided doses up to 24 mg/day; IM: 5-10 mg q6h as necessary up to 15-30 mg/day; IV (severe): 1 mg at 1- to 2-minute intervals up to a total of 5 mg. L.

Prochlorperazine (*Compazine*): [Capsule, sustained action: 10, 15, 30 mg; injection: 5 mg/mL; suppository: 2.5, 5.25 mg; syrup: 5 mg/5 mL; tablet: 5, 10, 25 mg]. Oral/IM: 5-10 mg 3-4 times/day; usual maximum: 40 mg/day; IV: 2.5-10 mg; maximum 10 mg/dose or 40 mg/day; may repeat dose q3-4h as needed; rectal: 25 mg twice daily. L.

Promazine (*Sparine*): [Injection: 25, 50 mg/mL; tablet: 25, 50, 100 mg]. Oral/IM: 25-50 mg q4-6h as needed. L.

Promethazine (*Phenergan*): [Injection: 25, 50 mg/mL; suppository: 12.5, 25, 50 mg; syrup: 6.25, 25 mg/5 mL; tablet: 12.5, 25, 50 mg]. Antiemetic: Oral, IM, IV, rectal: 12.5-25 mg q4h as needed; motion sickness: Oral, rectal: 25 mg 30-60 minutes before departure, then q12h as needed. L.

Thiethylperazine (*Norzine*): [Injection: 5 mg/mL; suppository: 10 mg; tablet: 10 mg]. Oral, IM, rectal: 10 mg 1-3 times/day as needed. L.

Trimethobenzamide (*Tigan*): [Capsule: 100, 250 mg; injection: 100 mg/mL; suppository: 100, 200 mg]. Oral: 250 mg 3-4 times/day; IM, rectal: 200 mg 3-4 times/day. L.

Antidiarrheals

Attapulgite (*Kaopectate*): [Liquid, oral concentrate: 600, 750 mg/15 mL; tablet: 750 mg; tablet, chewable: 300 mg, 600 mg]. 1200-1500 mg after each loose bowel movement or q2h; 15-30 mL up to 8 times/day, up to 9000 mg/24 hours. Not absorbed.

Bismuth subsalicylate (*Pepto-Bismol*): [Liquid, as subsalicylate: 262, 524 mg/15 mL, 240 mL; tablet: Chewable, as subsalicylate: 262 mg; chewable, as subgallate: 200 mg]. 2 tablets or 30 mL q30m to 1 hour as needed up to 8 doses/24 hours.

Diphenoxylate with atropine (*Lomotil*): [Solution, oral: Diphenoxylate hydrochloride 2.5 mg and atropine sulfate 0.025 mg/5 mL; tablet: Diphenoxylate hydrochloride 2.5 mg and atropine sulfate 0.025 mg]. 15-20 mg/day of diphenoxylate in 3-4 divided doses; maintenance: 5-15 mg/day in 2-3 divided doses. L.

Loperamide (*Imodium A-D*): [Caplet: 2 mg; capsule: 2 mg; liquid, oral: 1 mg/5 mL; tablet: 2 mg]. Initial: 4 mg (2 capsules), followed by 2 mg after each loose stool, up to 16 mg/day (8 capsules). L.

Antitussives/Expectorants

Benzonatate (*Tessalon Perles*): [100]. 100 mg PO tid. L.
Dextromethorphan (*Benylin DM*): [10 mg/5 mL]. 10-30 mg PO q4-8h. L.
Guaifenesin (*Robitussin*): [100 mg/5 mL]. 5-20 mL PO q4h. L.
Histussin HC [hydrocodone 2.5 mg + phenylephrine 5 mg + chlorpheniramine 2 mg/5 mL]. 10 mL q4h up to 40 mL/day.
Hydrocodone (*Hycodan*): 5 mL PO q4-6h. L.
Terpin hydrate: [elixir 85 mg/5 mL]. 5-10 mL PO tid/qid. L.

125

ASSESSMENT INSTRUMENTS

Mini-Mental State Examination (MMSE)

Add points for each correct response.

		Score	Points
Orientation			
1. What is the:	Year?	___	1
	Season?	___	1
	Date?	___	1
	Day?	___	1
	Month?	___	1
2. Where are we?	State?	___	1
	County?	___	1
	Town or city?	___	1
	Hospital?	___	1
	Floor?	___	1

Registration

3. Name three objects, taking 1 second to say each. Then ask the patient to repeat all three after you have said them.   ___   3

Give one point for each correct answer. Repeat the answers until patient learns all three.

Attention and calculation

4. Serial sevens. Give one point for each correct answer. Stop after five answers. Alternate: Spell WORLD backwards.   ___   5

Recall

5. Ask for names of three objects learned in question 3. Give one point for each correct answer.   ___   3

Language

6. Point to a pencil and a watch. Have the patient name them as you point.   ___   2

7. Have the patient repeat "No ifs, ands, or buts."   ___   1

8. Have the patient follow a three-stage command: "Take a paper in your right hand. Fold the paper in half. Put the paper on the floor."   ___   3

9. Have the patient read and obey the following: "CLOSE YOUR EYES." (Write it in large letters.)   ___   1

10. Have the patient write a sentence of his or her choice. (The sentence should contain a subject and an object and should make sense. Ignore spelling errors when scoring.)   ___   1

11. Have the patient copy the design. (Give one point if all sides and angles are preserved and if the intersecting sides form a quadrangle.)   ___   1

___ = Total 30

SOURCE: Courtesy of Marshal F. Folstein, MD. Reprinted with permission.

For additional information on administration and scoring, refer to the following references:

1. Folstein MF, Folstein S, McHugh PR. Mini-Mental State: a practical method for grading the cognitive state of patients for the clinician. *J Psychiatr Res.* 1975;12:189–198.
2. Tombaugh TN, McIntyre NJ. The Mini-Mental State Examination: a comprehensive review. *J Am Geriatr Soc.* 1992;40(9):922–935.

Activities of Daily Living (ADL) Scale Evaluation Form

Name_____ Day of evaluation_____

For each area of functioning listed below, check description that applies. (The word "assistance" means supervision, direction, or personal assistance.)

Bathing—either sponge bath, tub bath, or shower

☐	☐	☐
Receives no assistance (gets in and out of tub by self, if tub is usual means of bathing)	Receives assistance in bathing only one part of the body (such as back or a leg)	Receives assistance in bathing more than one part of the body (or not bathed)

Dressing—gets clothes from closets and drawers, including underclothes, outer garments, and using fasteners (including braces, if worn)

☐	☐	☐
Gets clothes and gets completely dressed without assistance	Gets clothes and gets dressed without assistance, except for assistance in tying shoes	Receives assistance in getting clothes or in getting dressed, or stays partly or completely undressed

Toileting—going to the "toilet room" for bowel and urine elimination; cleaning self after elimination and arranging clothes

☐	☐	☐
Goes to "toilet room," cleans self, and arranges clothes without assistance (may use object for support such as cane, walker, or wheelchair and may manage night bedpan or commode, emptying same in morning)	Receives assistance in going to "toilet room" or in cleansing self or in arranging clothes after elimination or in use of night bedpan or commode	Doesn't go to room termed "toilet" for the elimination process

Transfer

☐	☐	☐
Moves in and out of bed as well as in and out of chair without assistance (may be using object for support, such as cane or walker)	Moves in and out of bed or chair with assistance	Doesn't get out of bed

Continence

☐	☐	☐
Controls urination and bowel movement completely by self	Has occasional "accidents"	Supervision helps keep urine or bowel control; catheter is used or person is incontinent

Feeding

☐	☐	☐
Feeds self without assistance	Feeds self except for getting assistance in cutting meat or buttering bread	Receives assistance in feeding or is fed partly or completely by using tubes or intravenous fluids

SOURCE: Courtesy of Sidney Katz, MD. Reprinted with permission.

For additional information on administration and scoring, refer to the following references:
1. Katz S. Assessing self-maintenance: activities of daily living, mobility, and instrumental activities of daily living. *J Am Geriatr Soc.* 1983;31:721–727.
2. Katz S, Akpom CA. A measure of primary sociobiologic functions. *Int J Health Serv.* 1976;6:493–508.
3. Katz S, Downs TD, Cash HR, et al. Progress in development of the index of ADL. *J Gerontol.* 1970;10(1):20–30.

Instrumental Activities of Daily Living (IADL) Scale

Self-Rated Version Extracted from the Multilevel Assessment Instrument (MAI)

1. **Can you use the telephone:**
   without help, — 3
   with some help, or — 2
   are you completely unable to use the telephone? — 1

2. **Can you get to places out of walking distance:**
   without help, — 3
   with some help, or — 2
   are you completely unable to travel unless special arrangements are made? — 1

3. **Can you go shopping for groceries:**
   without help, — 3
   with some help, or — 2
   are you completely unable to do any shopping? — 1

4. **Can you prepare your own meals:**
   without help, — 3
   with some help, or — 2
   are you completely unable to prepare any meals? — 1

5. **Can you do your own housework:**
   without help, — 3
   with some help, or — 2
   are you completely unable to do any housework? — 1

6. **Can you do your own handyman work:**
   without help, — 3
   with some help, or — 2
   are you completely unable to do any handyman work? — 1

7. **Can you do your own laundry:**
   without help, — 3
   with some help, or — 2
   are you completely unable to do any laundry at all? — 1

8a. **Do you take medicines or use any medications?**
   (If yes, answer Question 8b) Yes — 1
   (If no, answer Question 8c) No — 2

8b. **Do you take your own medicine:**
   without help (in the right doses at the right time), — 3
   with some help (take medicine if someone prepares it for you and/or reminds you to take it), — 2
   or (are you/would you be) completely unable to take your own medicine? — 1

8c. **If you had to take medicine, can you do it:**
   without help (in the right doses at the right time), — 3
   with some help (take medicine if someone prepares it for you and/or reminds you to take it), — 2
   or (are you/would you be) completely unable to take your own medicine? — 1

9. **Can you manage your own money:**
   without help, — 3
   with some help, or — 2
   are you completely unable to handle money? — 1

SOURCE: Lawton MP, Brody EM. Assessment of older people: self-maintaining and instrumental activities of daily living. *The Gerontologist*. 1969;9:179–185. Copyright © The Gerontological Society of America. Reprinted with permission.

For additional information on administration and scoring, refer to the following references:
1. Lawton MP. Scales to measure competence in everyday activities. *Psychopharmacol Bull.* 1988;24(4):609–614.
2. Lawton MP, Moss M, Fulcomer M, et al. A research and service-oriented Multilevel Assessment Instrument.. *J Gerontol.* 1982;37:91–99.

Geriatric Depression Scale (short form)

Choose the best answer for how you felt over the past week.

1. Are you basically satisfied with your life?   yes/NO

2. Have you dropped many of your activities and interests?   YES/no

3. Do you feel that your life is empty?   YES/no

4. Do you often get bored?   YES/no

5. Are you in good spirits most of the time?   yes/NO

6. Are you afraid that something bad is going to happen to you?   YES/no

7. Do you feel happy most of the time?   yes/NO

8. Do you often feel helpless?   YES/no

9. Do you prefer to stay at home, rather than going out and doing new things?   YES/no

10. Do you feel you have more problems with memory than most?   YES/no

11. Do you think it is wonderful to be alive now?   yes/NO

12. Do you feel pretty worthless the way you are now?   YES/no

13. Do you feel full of energy?   yes/NO

14. Do you feel that your situation is hopeless?   YES/no

15. Do you think that most people are better off than you are?   YES/no

This is the scoring for the scale. One point for each response that is in capital letters.
Cut-off: normal (0–5), above 5 suggests depression.

SOURCE: Courtesy of Jerome A. Yesavage, MD. Reprinted with permission.

For additional information on administration and scoring, refer to the following references:
1. Sheikh JI, Yesavage JA. Geriatric Depression Scale: recent evidence and development of a shorter version. *Clin Gerontol.* 1986;5:165–172.
2. Yesavage JA, Brink TL, Rose TL, et al. Development and validation of a geriatric depression rating scale: a preliminary report. *J Psychiatr Res.* 1983;17:27.

Hearing Handicap Inventory for the Elderly (HHIE-S)

	Yes (4)	Sometimes (2)	No (0)
Does a hearing problem cause you to feel embarrassed when meeting new people?	____	____	____
Does a hearing problem cause you to feel frustrated when talking to members of your family?	____	____	____
Do you have difficulty hearing when someone speaks in a whisper?	____	____	____
Do you feel handicapped by a hearing problem?	____	____	____
Does a hearing problem cause you difficulty when visiting friends, relatives, or neighbors?	____	____	____
Does a hearing problem cause you to attend religious services less often than you would like?	____	____	____
Does a hearing problem cause you to have arguments with family members?	____	____	____
Does a hearing problem cause you difficulty when listening to TV or radio?	____	____	____
Do you feel that any difficulty with your hearing limits or hampers your personal or social life?	____	____	____
Does a hearing problem cause you difficulty when in a restaurant with relatives or friends?	____	____	____

Note: Range of total points, 0-40; 0-8, no self-perceived handicap; 10-22, mild to moderate handicap; 24-40, significant handicap.

Source: Ventry IM, Weinstein BE. Identification of elderly people with hearing problems. *ASHA.* 1983;25:37–42. ©American Speech-Language-Hearing Association. Reprinted by permission.

BALANCE
Chair
Instructions: Place a hard armless chair against a wall. The following maneuvers are tested.

1. **Sitting down**
   - 0 = unable without help *or* collapses (plops) into chair *or* lands off center of chair
   - 1 = able and does not meet criteria for 0 or 2
   - 2 = sits in a smooth, safe motion *and* ends with buttocks against back of chair and thighs centered on chair

2. **Sitting balance**
   - 0 = unable to maintain position (marked slide forward or leans forward or to side)
   - 1 = leans in chair slightly or slight increased distance from buttocks to back of chair
   - 2 = steady, safe, upright

3. **Arising**
   - 0 = unable without help or loses balance or requires > three attempts
   - 1 = able but requires three attempts
   - 2 = able in ≤ two attempts

4. **Immediate standing balance (first 5 seconds)**
   - 0 = unsteady, marked staggering, moves feet, marked trunk sway or grabs object for support
   - 1 = steady but uses walker or cane *or* mild staggering but catches self without grabbing object
   - 2 = steady without walker or cane or other support

Stand
5a. **Side-by-side standing balance**
   - 0 = unable *or* unsteady *or* holds ≤3 seconds
   - 1 = able *but* uses cane, walker or other support *or* holds for 4 to 9 seconds
   - 2 = narrow stance without support for 10 seconds

5b. **Timing ___ ___. ___ seconds**

6. **Pull test (subject at maximum position attained in #5, examiner stands behind and exerts mild pull back at waist)**
   - 0 = begins to fall
   - 1 = takes more than two steps back
   - 2 = fewer than two steps backward and steady

7a. **Able to stand on right leg unsupported**
   - 0 = unable *or* holds onto any object *or* able for <3 seconds
   - 1 = able for 3 or 4 seconds
   - 2 = able for 5 seconds

7b. **Timing ___ ___. ___ seconds**

8a. **Able to stand on left leg unsupported**
   - 0 = unable *or* holds onto any object *or* able for <3 seconds
   - 1 = able for 3 or 4 seconds
   - 2 = able for 5 seconds

8b. **Timing ___ ___. ___ seconds**

9a. **Semitandem stand**
   - 0 = unable to stand with one foot half in front of other with feet touching *or* begins to fall *or* holds for ≤3 seconds
   - 1 = able for 4 to 9 seconds
   - 2 = able to semitandem stand for 10 seconds

9b. **Timing ___ ___. ___ seconds**

131

10a. Tandem stand
0 = unable to stand with one foot in front of other *or* begins to fall *or* holds for ≤3 seconds
1 = able for 4 to 9 seconds
2 = able to tandem stand for 10 seconds

10b. Timing ___ ___ . ___ seconds

11. Bending over (to pick up a pen off floor)
0 = unable *or* is unsteady
1 = able, but requires more than one attempt to get up
2 = able and is steady

12. Toe stand
0 = unable
1 = able but <3 seconds
2 = able for 3 seconds

13. Heel stand
0 = unable
1 = able but <3 seconds
2 = able for 3 seconds

Bed or Couch
14. Stand to sit
0 = unable without help *or* collapses (plops) onto bed *or* falls back onto side *or* lands
   close to edge of bed
1 = able and does not meet criteria for 0 or 2
2 = able in a smooth motion *and* ends with buttocks away from edge of bed

15. Sit to lie
0 = unable without help *or* lands close to edge of bed *or* > three attempts
1 = able but requires three attempts
2 = able in ≤ two attempts

16. Lie to sit
0 = unable without help *or* ≥ three attempts *or* ends close to edge
1 = able but requires three attempts (falls back, or getting legs over)
2 = able in ≤ two attempts

17. Sit to stand
0 = unable without help *or* loses balance *or* requires > three attempts
1 = able but requires three attempts
2 = able in ≤ two attempts

Possible score: 36 [18 not included in scoring]

18. Was the transfer to and from:
1 = bed
2 = couch

GAIT
Instructions: Subject stands with examiner. Walks down 10- foot walkway (measured). Ask subject to
walk down walkway, turn, and walk back. Subject should use customary walking aid.

Bare Floor (flat, even surface)
1. Type of surface: 1 = linoleum/tile; 2 = wood; 3 = cement/concrete; 4 = other _____
   [not included in scoring]

2. Initiation of gait (immediately after told to "go")
0 = any hesitancy or multiple attempts to start
1 = no hesitancy

3. **Path** (estimated in relation to *tape measure*). Observe excursion of foot closest to tape measure over middle eight feet of course.

   0 = marked deviation
   1 = mild/moderate deviation *or* uses walking aid
   2 = straight without walking aid

4. **Missed step** (trip or loss of balance)

   0 = yes and would have fallen *or* more than two missed steps
   1 = yes, but appropriate attempt to recover *and* no more than two
   2 = none

5. **Turning** (while walking)

   0 = almost falls
   1 = mild staggering but catches self, uses walker or cane
   2 = steady, without walking aid

6. **Step over obstacles** (to be assessed in a separate walk with two shoes placed on course four feet apart)

   0 = begins to fall at any obstacle *or* unable to walks around any obstacle *or* > two missed steps
   1 = able to step over all obstacles but some staggering but catches self *or* one to two missed steps
   2 = able and steady at stepping over all four obstacles with no missed steps

Uneven or Thick Surface—choose in order below:

1. **1 = thick carpet; 2 = grass; 3 = thin carpet** [not included in scoring]

2. **Initiation of gait** (immediately after told to "go")

   0 = any hesitancy or multiple attempts to start
   1 = no hesitancy

3. **Path** (estimated in relation to *tape measure*). Observe excursion of foot closest to tape measure over middle eight feet of course

   0 = marked deviation
   1 = mild/moderate deviation *or* uses walking aid
   2 = straight without walking aid

4. **Missed step** (trip or loss of balance)

   0 = yes and would have fallen *or* more than two missed steps
   1 = yes, but appropriate attempt to recover *and* no more than two
   2 = none

5. **Turning** (while walking)

   0 = almost falls
   1 = mild staggering but catches self, uses walker or cane
   2 = steady without walking aid

6. **Step over obstacles** (to be assessed in a separate walk with two shoes placed on course)

   0 = begins to fall at any obstacle *or* unable, *or* walks around any obstacle *or* > two missed steps
   1 = able to step over all obstacles but some staggering but catches self *or* one to two missed steps
   2 = able and steady at stepping over all four obstacles with no missed steps

Possible score: 18

SOURCE: Courtesy of Mary E. Tinetti, MD. Reprinted with permission.

Examination Procedure

Either before or after completing the Examination Procedure, observe the patient
unobtrusively, at rest (eg, in waiting room).

The chair to be used in this examination should be a hard, firm one without arms.

1. Ask patient to remove shoes and socks.

2. Ask patient whether there is anything in his/her mouth (ie, gum, candy, etc) and if there is, to remove it.

3. Ask patient about the **current** condition of his/her teeth. Ask patient if he/she wears dentures.
   Do teeth or dentures bother patient **now**?

4. Ask patient whether he/she notices any movements in mouth, face, hands, or feet. If yes, ask to
   describe and to what extent they **currently** bother patient or interfere with his/her activities.

5. Have patient sit in chair with hands on knees, legs slightly apart, and feet flat on floor. (Look at entire
   body for movements while in this position.)

6. Ask patient to sit with hands hanging unsupported. If male, between legs, if female and wearing a
   dress, hanging over knees. (Observe hands and other body areas.)

7. Ask patient to open mouth. (Observe tongue at rest within mouth.) Do this twice.

8. Ask patient to protrude tongue. (Observe abnormalities of tongue movement) Do this twice.

9. Ask patient to tap thumb with each finger as rapidly as possible for 10 to 15 seconds; separately with
   right hand, then with left hand. (Observe facial and leg movements.)

10. Flex and extend patient's left and right arms (one at a time). (Note any rigidity.)

11. Ask patient to stand up. (Observe in profile. Observe all body areas again, hips included.)

12. Ask patient to extend both arms outstretched in front with palms down. (Observe trunk, legs,
    and mouth.)

13. Have patient walk a few paces, turn, and walk back to chair. (Observe hands and gait.) Do this twice.

Instructions: Complete examination procedure before making ratings. Rate highest severity observed.
Code: 1   None
       2   Minimal, may be extreme normal
       3   Mild
       4   Moderate
       5   Severe

Facial and Oral Movements

1. Muscles of facial expression (eg, movements of forehead, eyebrows, periorbital area, cheeks;
   including frowning, blinking, smiling, grimacing)
       1   2   3   4   5

2. Lips and perioral area (eg, puckering, pouting, smacking)
       1   2   3   4   5

3. Jaw (eg, biting, clenching, chewing, mouth opening, lateral movement)
       1   2   3   4   5

4. Tongue (rate only increase in movement both in and out of mouth, NOT inability to sustain movement)
       1   2   3   4   5

Extremity Movements

5. Upper (arms, wrists, hands, fingers). Include choreic movements (ie, rapid, objectively purposeless, irregular, spontaneous), athetoid movements (ie, slow, irregular, complex, serpentine). Do NOT include tremor (ie, repetitive, regular, rhythmic).

      1   2   3   4   5

6. Lower (legs, knees, ankles, toes). (eg, lateral knee movement, foot tapping, heel dropping, foot squirming, inversion and eversion of foot).

      1   2   3   4   5

Trunk Movements

7. Neck, shoulders, hips (eg, rocking, twisting, squirming, pelvic gyrations)

      1   2   3   4   5

Global Judgments

8. Severity of abnormal movements
   1. None, normal
   2. Minimal
   3. Mild
   4. Moderate
   5. Severe

9. Incapacitation due to abnormal movements
   1. None, normal
   2. Minimal
   3. Mild
   4. Moderate
   5. Severe

10. Patient's awareness of abnormal movements (rate only patient's report)
    1. No awareness
    2. Aware, no distress
    3. Aware, mild distress
    4. Aware, moderate distress
    5. Aware, severe distress

Dental Status

11. Current problems with teeth and/or dentures
    1. No
    2. Yes

12. Does patient usually wear dentures?
    1. No
    2. Yes

SOURCE: Adapted from *Treatment Strategies in Schizophrenia*. Washington, DC: Department of Health and Human Services, Public Health Service, Alcohol, Drug Abuse and Mental Health Administration, National Institute of Mental Health. ADM-117. Revised 1985.

© The Regents of the University of Michigan, 1991

		Yes (1)	No (0)
1.	After drinking have you ever noticed an increase in your heart rate or beating in your chest?	1. ___	___
2.	When talking with others, do you ever underestimate how much you actually drink?	2. ___	___
3.	Does alcohol make you sleepy so that you often fall asleep in your chair?	3. ___	___
4.	After a few drinks, have you sometimes not eaten or been able to skip a meal because you don't feel hungry?	4. ___	___
5.	Does having a few drinks help decrease your shakiness or tremors?	5. ___	___
6.	Does alcohol sometimes make it hard for you to remember parts of the day or night?	6. ___	___
7.	Do you have rules for yourself that you won't drink before a certain time of day or night?	7. ___	___
8.	Have you lost interest in hobbies or activities you used to enjoy?	8. ___	___
9.	When you wake up in the morning, do you ever have trouble remembering part of the night before?	9. ___	___
10.	Does having a drink help you sleep?	10. ___	___
11.	Do you hide your alcohol bottles from family members?	11. ___	___
12.	After a social gathering, have you ever felt embarrassed because you drank too much?	12. ___	___
13.	Have you ever been concerned that drinking might be harmful to your health?	13. ___	___
14.	Do you like to end an evening with a nightcap?	14. ___	___
15.	Did you find your drinking increased after someone close to you died?	15. ___	___
16.	In general, would you prefer to have a few drinks at home rather than go out to social events?	16. ___	___
17.	Are you drinking more now than in the past?	17. ___	___
18.	Do you usually take a drink to relax or calm your nerves?	18. ___	___
19.	Do you drink to take your mind off your problems?	19. ___	___
20.	Have you ever increased your drinking after experiencing a loss in your life?	20. ___	___
21.	Do you sometimes drive when you have had too much to drink?	21. ___	___
22.	Has a doctor or nurse ever said they were worried or concerned about your drinking?	22. ___	___
23.	Have you ever made rules to manage your drinking?	23. ___	___
24.	When you feel lonely does having a drink help?	24. ___	___

Scoring: 5 or more "yes" responses indicative of alcohol problem.

Source: Regents of the University of Michigan; 1991. Reprinted with permission.

For further information, contact Frederic Blow, PhD, University of Michigan Alcohol Research Center, 400 E. Eisenhower Parkway, Suite A, Ann Arbor, MI 48104, (734) 998-7952.

10-minute Screener for Geriatric Conditions		
Problem	**Screening Measure**	**Positive Screen**
Vision	Two parts: Ask: "Do you have difficulty driving or watching television or reading or doing any of your daily activities because of your eyesight?" If yes, then: Test each eye with Snellen chart while patient wears corrective lenses (if applicable).	Yes to question and inability to read greater than 20/40 on Snellen chart.
Hearing	Use audioscope set at 40 dB. Test hearing using 1000 and 2000 Hz	Inability to hear 1000 or 2000 Hz in both ears; or inability to hear frequencies in either ear.
Leg mobility	Time the patient after asking: "Rise from the chair. Walk 20 feet briskly, turn, walk back to the chair and sit down."	Unable to complete task in 15 seconds.
Urinary incontinence	Two parts: Ask: "In the past year, have you ever lost your urine and gotten wet?" If yes, then ask: "Have you lost urine on at least 6 separate days?"	Yes to both questions.
Nutrition, weight loss	Two parts Ask: "Have you lost 10 lbs over the past 6 months without trying to do so?" Weigh the patient.	Yes to the question or weight < 100 lb.
Memory	Three-item recall.	Unable to remember all three items after 1 minute.
Depression	Ask: "Do you often feel sad or depressed?"	Yes to the question.
Physical disability	Six questions: "Are you able to . . . "Do strenuous activities like fast walking or bicycling?" "Do heavy work around the house like washing windows, walls, or floors?" "Go shopping for groceries or clothes?" "Get to places out of walking distance?" "Bathe, either a sponge bath, tub bath, or shower?" "Dress, like putting on a shirt, buttoning and zipping, or putting on shoes?"	Yes to any of the questions.

Source: Adapted from Moore AA, Siu AL. Screening for common problems in ambulatory elderly: clinical confirmation of a screen instrument. *Am J Med.* 1996;100:440. Permission to reprint.

OBRA REGULATIONS

Antidepressants

Drug	Brand Name	Usual Max Daily Dose for Age ≥65	Usual Max Daily Dose
Amitriptyline	Elavil®	150 mg	300 mg
Amoxapine	Asendin®	200 mg	400 mg
Desipramine	Norpramin®	150 mg	300 mg
Doxepin	Adapin®, Sinequan®	150 mg	300 mg
Imipramine	Tofranil®	150 mg	300 mg
Maprotiline	Ludiomil®	150 mg	300 mg
Nortriptyline	Aventyl®, Pamelor®	75 mg	150 mg
Protriptyline	Vivactil®	30 mg	60 mg
Trazodone	Desyrel®	300 mg	600 mg
Trimipramine	Surmontil®	150 mg	300 mg

Antipsychotic Medication Guidelines

Appropriate indications for use of antipsychotic medications are outlined in the Health Care Finance Administration's Omnibus Reconciliation Act (OBRA) of 1987. In addition to psychotic disorders, specific nonpsychotic behavior is identified for antipsychotic treatment. Specifically, behavior associated with organic mental syndromes (nonpsychotic behavior) is indicated:

- Agitated psychotic symptoms (biting, kicking, hitting, scratching, assertive and belligerent behavior, sexual aggressiveness) that present a danger to themselves or others or interfere with family and/or staff's ability to provide care (activities of daily living [ADL])
- Psychotic symptoms (hallucinations, delusions, paranoia)
- Continuous (24-hour) crying out and screaming

Behavior less responsive to antipsychotic therapy includes:
- Repetitive, bothersome behavior (ie, pacing, wandering, repeated statements or words, calling out, fidgeting)
- Poor self-care
- Unsociability
- Indifference to surroundings
- Uncooperative behavior
- Restlessness
- Impaired memory
- Anxiety
- Depression
- Insomnia

If antipsychotic therapy is to be used for one or more of these symptoms only, then the use of antipsychotic agents is inappropriate. Antipsychotic agents may worsen these symptoms, especially symptoms of sedation and lethargy, as well as enhance "confusion" due to their anticholinergic properties.

Selection of an antipsychotic agent should be based on the side-effect profile since all antipsychotic agents are equally effective at equivalent doses. Coadministration of two or more antipsychotics does not have any pharmacologic basis or clinical advantage. Coadministration of two or more antipsychotic agents does not improve clinical response and increases the potential for side effects.

Once behavior control is obtained, assess patient to determine if precipitating event (stress from drugs, fluid/electrolyte changes, infection, changes in environment) has been resolved or patient has accommodated to the environment or situation. Determine whether the antipsychotic can be decreased in dose or tapered off completely by monitoring selected target symptoms for which the antipsychotic therapy was initiated. OBRA '87 requires attempts at dose reduction within a 6-month period unless documented as to why this cannot be done. Identifying target symptoms is essential for adequate monitoring. Due to side effects, intermittent use (not PRN) is preferable (ie, only when patient has behavior warranting use of these agents). See also Federal OBRA Regulations Antipsychotics chart in this Appendix.

Antipsychotics				
Drug	Brand Name	Usual Max Daily Dose for Age ≥65	Usual Max Daily Dose	Daily Oral Dose for Residents With Organic Mental Syndromes
Acetophenazine	Tindal®	150 mg	300 mg	20 mg
Chlorpromazine	Thorazine®	800 mg	1600 mg	75 mg
Chlorprothixene	Taractan®	800 mg	1600 mg	75 mg
Clozapine	Clozaril®	25 mg	450 mg	50 mg
Fluphenazine	Prolixin®	20 mg	40 mg	4 mg
Haloperidol	Haldol®	50 mg	100 mg	4 mg
Loxapine	Loxitane®	125 mg	250 mg	10 mg
Mesoridazine	Serentil®	250 mg	500 mg	25 mg
Molindone	Moban®	112 mg	225 mg	10 mg
Perphenazine	Trilafon®	32 mg	64 mg	8 mg
Promazine	Sparine®	50 mg	500 mg	150 mg
Risperidone	Risperdal®	1 mg	16 mg	4 mg
Thioridazine	Mellaril®	400 mg	800 mg	75 mg
Thiothixene	Navane®	30 mg	60 mg	7 mg
Trifluoperazine	Stelazine®	40 mg	80 mg	8 mg
Trifluopromazine	Vesprin®	100 mg	20 mg	–

Anxiolytic Therapy Guidelines

The use of anxiolytics is acceptable as long as other disease processes that could explain anxious behavior have been ruled out. Daily use, at any dose, is for less than 4 continuous months, unless an attempt at dose reduction is unsuccessful. Proper indications include:

- Generalized anxiety disorder
- Organic mental syndrome (including dementia associated with agitation)
- Panic disorders
- Anxiety associated with other psychiatric disorder (eg, depression, adjustment disorder)

Anxiolytics*			
Drug	Brand Name	Usual Max Daily Dose for Age ≥65	Usual Daily Dose for Age <65
Alprazolam	Xanax®	2 mg	4 mg
Clorazepate	Tranxene®	30 mg	60 mg
Chlordiazepoxide	Librium®	40 mg	100 mg
Diazepam	Valium®	20 mg	60 mg
Halazepam	Paxipam®	80 mg	160 mg
Lorazepam	Ativan®	3 mg	6 mg
Meprobamate	Miltown®	600 mg	1600 mg
Oxazepam	Serax®	60 mg	90 mg
Prazepam	Centrax®	30 mg	60 mg

*Note: HCFA-OBRA guidelines strongly urge clinicians not to use barbiturates, glutethimide, and ethchlorvynol due to their side effects, pharmacokinetics, and addiction potential in the elderly. Also, HCFA discourages use of long-acting benzodiazepines in the elderly.

Hypnotic Therapy Guidelines

Hypnotics are allowed for 10 continuous days of use. If three unsuccessful attempts at dose reduction occur, then it is clinically contraindicated to reduce.

Drug	Brand Name	Usual Max Single Dose for Age ≥65	Usual Max Single Dose for Age <65
Alprazolam	Xanax®	0.25 mg	1.5 mg
Amobarbital	Amytal®	105 mg	300 mg
Butabarbital	Butisol®	100 mg	200 mg
Chloral hydrate	Noctec®	750 mg	1500 mg
Chloral hydrate	Various	500 mg	1000 mg
Diphenhydramine	Benadryl®	25 mg	50 mg
Ethchlorvynol	Placidyl®	500 mg	1000 mg
Flurazepam	Dalmane®	15 mg	30 mg
Glutethimide	Doriden®	500 mg	1000 mg
Halazepam	Paxipam®	20 mg	40 mg
Hydroxyzine	Atarax®	50 mg	100 mg
Lorazepam	Ativan®	1 mg	2 mg
Methyprylon	Noludar®	200 mg	400 mg
Oxazepam	Serax®	15 mg	30 mg
Phenobarbital	Nembutal®	100 mg	200 mg
Secobarbital	Seconal®	100 mg	200 mg*
Temazepam	Restoril®	15 mg	30 mg
Triazolam	Halcion®	0.125 mg	0.5 mg

*Note: HCFA-OBRA guidelines strongly urge clinicians not to use barbiturates, glutethimide, and ethchlorvynol due to their side effects, pharmacokinetics, and addiction potential in the elderly. Also, HCFA discourages use of long-acting benzodiazepines in the elderly.

SUBJECT INDEX

(The letter "t" after a page number indicates a Table)